For Andy!
with best wishes for
adventures of your own.

On the Ledge

On the Ledge

A Doctor's Stories from the Inner City

NEIL S. SKOLNIK, M.D.

Faber and Faber

BOSTON • LONDON

Excerpt from "Musee des Beaux Arts" from *W. H. Auden: Collected
Poems* by W. H. Auden. Copyright © 1940 and renewed 1968 by
W. H. Auden. Reprinted by permission of Random House, Inc.

Library of Congress Cataloging-in-Publication Data

Skolnik, Neil
   On the ledge : a doctor's stories from the inner city / Neil Skolnik.
     p. cm.
   ISBN 0-571-19883-X (cloth)
   1. Urban poor—Medical care—United States. I. Title.
  RA418.5.P6S595   1996
  362.1'0425—dc20   95-39071
                                                    CIP

Jacket design by Peter Blaiwas
Jacket photograph from the collection of the author
Printed in the United States of America

This book is dedicated to

ARTHUR AND JINNY SKOLNIK,
who taught me the value of hard work,
honesty, dedication, and joy

ALISON SKOLNIK,
who taught and teaches me
the value of love,
sensitivity, and feeling

HEIDI SKOLNIK,
who keeps my values system
straight

AARON AND AVA,
who are
my future

There are no answers,
seek them lovingly.

—THE TALMUD

Contents

Acknowledgments

A book is brought to fruition with the help of many people. These people deserve acknowledgment:

My patients, who taught me about their lives and who trusted me to take care of them.

David Slavitt, an accomplished poet and novelist, who was generous as a mentor in writing and whose confidence, friendship, and incredibly critical and honest approach taught me a great deal.

Steve Hollenberg, who read every chapter as it was written, who gave me feedback on every line, and who has the sharpest critical eye I can imagine;

Howard Rabinowitz, a friend and mentor who read many of the chapters and gave important critical feedback.

My mentors and colleagues in the family medicine residency program at Thomas Jefferson University Hospital, where I did my residency in family medicine. Much of what I know about medicine I learned there. Specific individuals who deserve special mention include: Paul Brucker, for serving as a role model of utmost integrity, caring, and hard work and for having given me the opportunity to work at the family medicine office that this book is about, as well as for sage advice over the last decade; Rich Wender, who taught me a great deal about medicine, about patients, and most importantly taught me that medicine is fun; and Bob Perkel, who taught me about patient care and supported the idea that medicine and literature are a good mix.

The staff and administration of Abington Memorial Hospital for their interest in, and encouragement of, my writing these stories, and for their support of the Family Medicine Residency Program that provides excellent, compassionate medical care to patients from a wide variety of social, cultural, and economic backgrounds.

Herb Adler, whose ideas on stories were elucidating; Todd Sagin, for constant support and for ideas shared; Dave Eskin, for his appreciation and encouragement of this project as well as for reading many of the stories prior to publication; Neil Schlackman, for helping to develop some important ideas; and Bea Drucker for her constant interest, encouragement, and support.

John Stone, for being a role model of an excellent clinician-educator-writer; Perri Klass, for a discussion over dinner, the time she took to read the manuscript, and her encouragement at a time when it was needed.

Cornelius Merlini, Kathy Clark, Mark Miles, and the people at Hoechst Marion Roussel for their excitement about the book, their concern about the health care of the urban poor, and their support of a project that allows this book to be given to first- and second-year medical students to be used in classrooms for learning about cross-cultural issues in the health care of the urban poor, addressing in a real way many of the issues raised in this book.

Roger Sherwood, Marjorie Bowmen, and the Society of Teachers of Family Medicine Foundation for their support and sponsorship of a project that will allow medical students to benefit from this book.

Anne Edelstein of the Anne Edelstein Literary Agency, for her help and persistence; Betsy Uhrig of Faber and Faber, for close and sensitive reading and editing of the manuscript; and Faber and Faber, for having the confidence and social concern to believe in this book enough to publish it.

Last and most importantly my wife, Alison, who was there the evening the first story in this book was conceived; who saw this manuscript develop from a purging of frustration into an article and then into a book; who read every chapter I wrote through almost every revision; who gave pointed, honest input and criticism that was sometimes difficult to hear but usually correct; who woke to drink coffee as I woke to write at five every morning for the first two years of our marriage, when my oversized desk was a foot and a half away from the foot of our bed in the first apartment we lived in together; who watched our children—first Aaron and then Aaron and Ava—while I typed; and who was, simply, supportive and encouraging, and who put up with my writing of this book during a time when we moved to three different homes, had two children, changed jobs and diapers, and shared innumerable other events too long, personal, and important to list. In addition, Alison came up with the first line of the book. To Alison, my love and appreciation.

Portions of this book have been previously published, as follows: "Ezekiel" was first published under the title "Failing to Thrive" in the *Philadelphia Inquirer Sunday Magazine*. "A Soft Snow Falling" was first published under the title "A Breathing Lesson" in *Philadelphia* magazine. "A Stitch in Time" was first published in *Archives of Family Medicine*.

All names, identifying characteristics, and other details of patients have been changed.

Introduction

Forthwith this frame of mine was wrenched
With a woeful agony,
Which forced me to begin my tale;
And then it left me free. . . .

And till my ghastly tale is told,
This heart within me burns.

> —SAMUEL TAYLOR COLERIDGE
> The Rime of the Ancient Mariner

IT IS THEIR HOME. These words echo in my mind at night. They are the first and last words in a short book that took five years to write. The events in this book occurred over a two-year period, from July 1987 to July 1989. I had just graduated from a three-year residency in family medicine, was full of idealism, and was well trained to handle the medical problems I would encounter.

The office described in this book was a well-run, small inner-city family medicine office. The office was located on the third floor of a four-story building and consisted of four examination rooms, a nurses' station, a small laboratory area with a microscope, and a consultation room with a window overlooking the surrounding community. Although patients were encouraged to make appointments, about half of the people who made appointments did not keep them, and about half of the patients we saw simply walked into the office without an appointment.

Most of the patients who came to the office had medical insurance provided to them through Medicaid, a program that provides insurance to people whose incomes fall below a predetermined line. Medicaid, in theory, should allow people to receive care who could not otherwise afford to get medical care. In fact, Medicaid pays physicians less for each patient visit than other type of insurance, and therefore many physicians do not treat patients who have Medicaid. This limits the choices and availability of medical care to poor patients. Many of our patients did not have any insurance. The cost of running the office was subsidized by the university that opened the office as part of its mission to serve the community.

The office was located in a run-down neighborhood about a block and a half from one of Philadelphia's large high-rise housing projects, which was about eight blocks from where I lived for five years. The differences between the neighborhood where I lived and the neighborhood where my patients lived should not have been a surprise, but was startling to me nonetheless. Each day as I would walk down the main thoroughfare from my home to our office, I would feel uncomfortable, and not completely safe, as I got to the two-block area closest to our office. This was the neighborhood where most of my patients lived.

The office provided family medicine services. Many people do not realize that family doctors still exist in the inner city. They do. Family doctors distinguish themselves by handling the full range of medical problems that occur in a community; this is true whether it is a rural community or the inner city. Family doctors care for children and adults, young and old, women and men, and they treat psychological as well as medical problems. They are trained to integrate knowledge from diverse fields of medicine to provide medical care in a comprehensive, personal, and consistent way. It has been said that in many specialties the disease is the constant phenomenon, which occurs to many patients over time. In family medicine, the patient is the constant phenomenon, who experiences and is treated for a number of diseases over time.

The wide range of medical care that can be provided by a family practitioner is an advantage in any medically underserved area such as the inner city. Most medical schools and hospitals realize the value of comprehensive care and have departments of family medicine. It remains puzzling why many large inner-city medical schools and hospitals still do not have departments of family medicine. These stories are written from the vantage point of a family practitioner, and so convey a sense of the compassion that most family doctors have for their patients as well as the breadth of problems that physicians see in the inner city.

Health Access in the United States

This book is about one office and one doctor. The events described, though, reflect the status of health care in cities across the country. Health care reform is an important political and economic issue. As the cost of health care in the

United States has skyrocketed, both the government and the business community have recognized that they must look for ways to control health care costs while expanding the provision of services to those who may not currently receive adequate health care. As we focus as a nation on the cost of health care, it is essential that we not lose sight of the people for whom that care is being—or, as the case may be, not being—provided.

Access to health care is a complex issue that crosses medical, social, cultural, and economic boundaries. There is no single cause of poor access to health care. Over the last ten years, research has shown that the health status of people in the inner city is significantly below that of other members of our society. As the reader takes part in the stories of the patients seen at our family medicine office, it is helpful to have in mind some of the differences in health outcomes between people who are poor and in the inner city and those of the rest of the nation.

In 1993 the Institute of Medicine published a monograph, *Access to Health Care in America,* that concluded that research into health care and health status shows "a growing division between the haves and the have-nots in our society." This, and a number of other studies, point out some troubling facts:

- People at the low end of the income scale have about half the contact with medical providers that others do.

- Admission rates to hospitals for conditions that should be controlled with appropriate outpatient care are on average four times higher for residents of low-income than high-income neighborhoods.

- In 1988, black infants were more than twice as likely as whites to die during their first year of life.

- For many chronic medical illnesses—such as congestive heart failure, hypertension, and asthma—for which appropriate outpatient care can often help avoid inpatient admission, there is a six- to sevenfold difference between the hospital admission rate for people living in low-income neighborhoods and those from high-income neighborhoods.

- Patients seen at centers that predominantly treat minorities are three times more likely than those treated elsewhere to have inadequate pain management.

- Ruptured appendix, a condition that is preventable when early medical care is obtained, is more likely among Medicaid and uninsured patients with appendicitis than among patients with private medical insurance.

- Immunization rates for children in the inner city are approximately 20 percent below those for children who live outside the city.

- Many contagious diseases are more common among people living in cities than among people living in other areas of the country; this is particularly true for people living in poor neighborhoods in the city. Specifically: the rate of tuberculosis is twice as high in Philadelphia as it is across the United States, and three times as high in poorer neighborhoods in Philadelphia as it is elsewhere; the rate of syphilis is almost five times as high in the inner city; the rate of gonorrhea is over three and a half times as high.

The Institute of Medicine concluded: "The most important consideration is whether people have the *opportunity* [emphasis added] for a good outcome—especially in those instances in which medical care can make a difference. When those opportunities are systematically denied to groups in society, there is an access problem that needs to be addressed."

As we pay attention to cost it is essential that we also pay attention to the human face of the health care that is being provided. Perhaps this book can help to give some perspective to complement the statistics to which we are commonly exposed. It will also become clear, in reading these stories, that access to health care in the inner city is more than simply having medical care available; true access involves creating a social structure that facilitates people's ability to receive medical care. It involves taking care of people.

Why Stories?

Although it is possible for the stories in this book to inform individuals about larger social issues, the main impulse for writing this book is more personal and much simpler—I felt a need to convey my experience to others about practicing medicine in the inner city. This reason for writing goes beyond any rationale I may now have for how these stories might be used or how they could influence the way others view complex issues of health care and access for the urban poor. The best way I know to convey my experience is through stories. Patients come to physicians with their stories, and physicians become participants in those stories. We all know this. We remember our parents, or aunts, or friends telling of their visits to the doctor.

Stories are one of the ways we have of organizing experience. Storytelling is also one of the methods by which we transform experience from something that can isolate us—by changing us in ways that other people may not understand—to something that brings us closer to others by creating bonds of shared understanding and feeling. It is ultimately, I suppose, this that I hope to accomplish: to create some shared understanding and feeling between myself and the reader of these stories.

August 1995

On the Ledge

IT IS THEIR HOME. From my office window I see the projects rise up out of the gutter, looming over the surrounding neighborhood. The neighborhood is filled with two- and three-story homes in disrepair, many with wooden boards over their windows. People living in this neighborhood come to my office for their medical care. They come in pain, they come crying, and they come hearing voices. They come after a tragedy in their family, a son killed in a drug war, a daughter addicted to cocaine. Some come because they feel lonely and need to talk. Others come short of breath. Some come with discharge, still others come vomiting blood. I patch what I can. I administer antibiotics; I give digitalis; I treat high blood pressure, diabetes, asthma, arthritis, congestive heart failure, syphilis, AIDS, and whatever else patients bring with them when they walk through the office door. I do fewer pap smears than I thought I would, and give fewer immunizations than I know I should. I sew up dripping wounds. As I sit looking out of the window at the end of the day, I find myself shaking.

I shake because I know how powerless I am to affect any of the things I see going on. Patients come into the office after drinking whiskey or shooting dope all weekend long, and I act as though I make a difference in their lives. If I were honest I could admit to them, and to myself, that the pills I prescribe for their high blood pressure have little chance of helping their true health problems. Their blood pressure alone is not going to kill them; their environment will. I tell them, though, to take their pills, trying to convince them that it will help their health, and often believing it myself. True, I advise them to stop drinking and to stop abusing drugs, but I know that if an individual has been drinking a pint of whiskey a day for the last twenty years, the chances of my changing this habit are extremely small.

I began working in this office this past July, after completing a three-year residency in family medicine. During my residency I was taught how to think about health and disease, how to diagnose medical and psychological problems, and how to treat people with illness. The training program I attended was an excellent one, and upon graduation I felt prepared to take care of patients on my own. During the last six months of my residency I interviewed a number of practices in an effort to find one that I wanted to work with. In late May an unexpected opening developed in an inner-city family medicine office operated by the same physicians I had trained under during residency, a group of excellent, socially concerned, caring physicians. I immediately applied for the job, and accepted it when it was offered. I felt that it would provide me with excellent medical experience as well as an opportunity to contribute medical care to an underserved community.

The prospect of practicing independently was exciting. I expected to learn a lot of medicine and to mature as a physician. This would be the first time in my career that

I would be the only one responsible for the care of my patients. There would be no one standing beside me, ready with advice when I needed it, as there always had been during medical school and residency. What I did not anticipate was how emotionally rending working with the urban poor would be, and what I would learn, in addition to medicine, about people, society, and myself.

This morning may have been the last time I will see Ralph Gregory. I started taking care of Mr. Gregory four months ago, shortly after I started working in this office, when he wandered in barely able to breathe. He did not have an appointment and I watched as the nurse led him down the hallway to the examination room. He was about fifty years old, had graying hair, and limped slightly as he walked. He appeared short of breath and sweating. When I examined him I found track marks up both his arms. Listening to his chest with my stethoscope I heard gurgling sounds, like the ones you hear when standing at the edge of a hot fountain at Yellowstone National Park the moment before boiling water shoots up through the rock. I placed my palm on his sticky chest and felt his heart pounding against his ribs as if it were a wild animal banging against a cage, trying to get out. His heart was at least twice the normal size, and through my stethoscope I heard murmurs and gallops, sounds that indicate advanced heart disease. Mr. Gregory's heart disease was most likely the result of years of excessive alcohol use, the alcohol eating away at the muscle of the heart as it does many other organs of the body. His heart was working hard, but it was still not pumping the blood his body needed, and as a consequence, his lungs were filling up with fluid. To improve his breathing, I admitted him to the hospital.

He did well during that hospital stay. We were able to get the fluid out of his lungs and by the time he left the hospital he was able to breathe comfortably. Mr. Gregory surprised me over the next two months by keeping his scheduled appointments every two weeks. During these visits I would listen to his heart and lungs, take his blood pressure, and adjust his medications. We would also discuss his heroin and alcohol addictions. He had tried to kick these habits a number of times by going though the city's detoxification programs. Shortly after leaving each program, he would start taking drugs again. Now, he told me, he was determined to break his addictions for good, and he would do it on his own. I was impressed that he was making an honest effort.

Two months after his discharge from the hospital he told me he was feeling nervous and jittery all the time and he didn't know why. He said he was scared that he was going to slip back into his old habits of using intravenous drugs. I suggested that he enroll in a drug abuse program but he didn't believe that it would work for him. He had been down that road too many times.

Mr. Gregory certainly had enough to be nervous about. His heart was in such bad shape that he was getting short of breath just walking down the hall; his years of intravenous drug abuse put him at risk of having AIDS; and his relationship with his girlfriend had deteriorated since his medical problems had begun to interfere with his ability to have erections. He asked if I would prescribe a "nerve pill," Alprazolam, that had helped him in the past.

The fact that he knew the name of the drug that he wanted prescribed concerned me. People with drug abuse problems often get addicted to anti-anxiety medications. I told him that if he agreed to return to the office every two weeks for counseling I would be willing to prescribe a two-week supply of Alprazolam at each office visit. During these counseling sessions we would discuss his substance abuse problem and I would give him what extra support I could. I hoped that this would help him stay away from intravenous drugs and allow me to make sure he was using the Alprazolam correctly. He agreed with this plan.

For two months it seemed as if my idea was working. Mr. Gregory kept his appointments. At these visits we would discuss both his medical and his social problems. He told me he was staying away from heroin and cocaine.

Last week he was an hour late for his appointment. The receptionist asked him to reschedule, but he insisted on being seen. When I walked into the examination room, Mr. Gregory couldn't sit still. Sweat was pouring from his face and he kept getting up from his chair, only to sit back down again. His voice was slurred and far too loud for the small examination room. He reminded me of a squirrel in the yard darting two feet to the right, stopping, then going back to the left again, every muscle in his body moving, ready to jump in any direction, but not going anywhere. He told me that he was feeling nervous, more nervous than usual, and needed more Alprazolam. He had run out of his medicine that morning.

He was not acting like himself, so I asked him if he had been doing any street drugs. He jumped up and his eyes bulged. "What you think I am?" His voice was filled with disdain and I felt, disappointment. I was letting him down, like all the other doctors and social workers he had ever dealt with. "Shhheeeiiit," his voice sounded like gravel rolling down a mountain, "What, you think I'm stupid? I ain't doin' no shit. What, you don't trust me no more?"

"It's not that I don't trust you, but . . ." I hesitated, not sure how to express my thoughts. I didn't trust him, with good reason. He appeared to be on speed, and he was at my office asking me to write a prescription for a drug that he might abuse. I felt like throwing him out. Instead I said, "I'd like to send a sample of urine to the lab and have it checked for drugs."

His fidgeting stopped as he stared at me, held out his hand, and said, "Give me the cup." He then went to the bathroom, returned a few minutes later with a urine specimen, placed it on the counter next to me, and walked out of the office.

The urine test revealed that he had heroin and cocaine in his system. What was not in his system was Alprazolam. For two months I had been writing prescriptions for anti-anxiety medication for Mr. Gregory, trusting that he was taking them to help combat his heroin addiction. Instead, as I later learned was fairly common among drug addicts, he was taking the prescription I gave him, obtaining the medicine for free using a medical card supplied to him by the city, and then selling the Alprazolam on the street for five to ten dollars a pill. The ninety pills I prescribed for him each month had a street value of almost one thousand dollars. He then used the money to support his heroin addiction. I had been taken.

This morning when he came into the office I discussed the results of his urine test with him. Then I told him that I would no longer prescribe Alprazolam for him.

"Bull," he said loudly, "the test's wrong. Send it again." He sounded as if he believed the next test would not show drugs in it.

"No," I said.

He shook his head, murmured "Shit," and walked out. I'm not sure if I'll ever see Mr. Gregory again. I do not expect him to come in now for his regular appointments. As he forgets to take his medicines his heart will get worse. Then, if he chooses to return to our office, it will be with his lungs filling with fluid, as it was the day we met.

It is often hard to make sense of what goes on in this office, but it goes on happening whether I understand it or not. I treat a woman for an infection in her fallopian tubes and I tell her that she has a sexually transmitted disease. I explain, as best as I can, the precautions she will need to take to avoid becoming infected again. She nods, and I give her a shot of an antibiotic. As I place the needle in the disposal container, I try to hide my irritation from the nurse, the patient, and at times from myself. I know there is a good chance that in the next few months I will see this woman again, walking into the office bent over in pain with another infection burning in her tubes, or worse. I know I am seeing only a small part of the problems my patients have and that the larger problems have nothing to do with medicine. The real problems have to do with environmental circumstances that I understand poorly and am powerless to change. All I can do is dispose of the syringe and move on to the next patient.

The next patient this afternoon was Ms. Bradley. Glancing at her chart before I walked in the room, I learned that Ms. Bradley was nineteen years old and had been seen two weeks before by my partner. My partner's note indicated that he was concerned about an ectopic, or tubal, pregnancy. An ectopic pregnancy occurs when a fertilized egg attaches to the fallopian tube and starts growing there instead of in the uterus. Since the fallopian tube has no room for a growing egg, it eventually bursts. As it bursts, dilated blood vessels that have grown around the developing embryo are ripped open, leading to massive bleeding into the abdominal cavity. Ectopic pregnancies can be difficult to diagnose early, before they can be detected with an ultrasound. Often the diagnosis can be made only by seeing whether a hormone that normally increases at a predictable rate during the course of a normal pregnancy does not increase as expected. My partner had drawn blood samples at the time he saw Ms. Bradley. He explained to her about the symptoms to watch for—abdominal pain and vaginal bleeding, which would mean she needed emergency medical care—and explained how dangerous an ectopic pregnancy can be without proper follow-up. He scheduled her to come back to the office the next day.

The blood samples that were drawn confirmed that Ms. Bradley was pregnant, but she did not keep her appointment. The nurse had called her home phone number, as it was written in the chart, but that number had been disconnected. The nurse then called Ms. Bradley's mother and left a message for the patient to come back into the office. My partner had also sent two registered letters to the patient emphasizing the importance of coming back in for medical care.

I walked into the room and found Ms. Bradley doubled over and sweating. She told me that her stomach hurt and that she was bleeding a lot from her vagina. She wanted a shot, she said, to make her feel better.

I asked her to lie down on the table and took her blood pressure. It was stable. I moved the gown from her abdomen and noticed that her skin looked like wrinkled seaweed, transformed from the supple young skin of a nineteen-year-old by her two prior pregnancies. Placing my hand, even lightly, on her belly caused her pain.

"Why you got to do that? Can't you jus' give me a shot?" she cried. I continued my exam. She was most tender over her right ovary. The pelvic exam confirmed an ectopic pregnancy.

The nurse called an ambulance while I called ahead to have a gynecologist meet her in the emergency room of the nearest hospital. A ruptured ectopic pregnancy can be fatal, and fast. The gynecologist confirmed the diagnosis and took Ms. Bradley immediately to the operating room, where she is now.

Marjeta Bradley is the same woman that I admitted to the hospital five months ago after she shot amphetamines into a vein in her arm while she was twelve weeks pregnant. That child aborted, probably because of those drugs. If she comes through the operation tonight, as I pray she will, we will have only patched things up for a very short time. Her main problems remain: her environment; her lack of ability to care for herself; her childhood, which ended with her first pregnancy when she was fourteen.

As I sit looking out my office window, what I find most disturbing as I think about the day, the thing that haunts me, is the look I saw in Ms. Bradley's eyes when I told her what was causing her pain. How little she seemed to care that a ruptured tube could kill her as well as the baby. How, when I told her that she would have to go to the hospital tonight for an operation, all I could feel from the look in her eyes was that I was inconveniencing her.

Ezekiel

"DON'T FORGET, THE PATIENT is the one with the illness," a graduating resident told me when I was a third-year medical student. The message was clear. As students and residents, we would have enough stress just dealing with long nights on call, our own feelings of inadequacy in taking care of patients, and our compulsion to learn about a patient's illness. There was no time to get entangled in their pain, which was a product of their illness, or to try to learn about their lives, which were often the cause of their illness. We would see patients during brief encounters, address their medical problems, and send them home.

Now, having practiced medicine for only six months in an office located a block from one of Philadelphia's largest housing projects, where I look out my office window and see a mother walking, holding her two-year-old son's hand, past a teenager handing a cellophane bag to a man in a beat-up car with out-of-state license plates, sayings such as the one above no longer seem conscionable, and they no longer serve their protective function. Many of the illnesses I see in this office are ones we have all created, and ones we all contribute to. To say that a five-month-old boy weighing eight pounds, lying on the examination table with skin clinging to bird-thin bones, staring out with blank eyes, is "the one with the illness" is absurd. We all have the illness. He is the one who has the symptoms.

Ezekiel's mother brought him to the office because he didn't look as bright or as big as her other five children had at the same age. Ezekiel's mother was twenty-three. When I walked into the room, she was sitting with Ezekiel lying across her lap. His foot was dangling down into the folds of her striped dress and his head hung over the outside of her thigh. Her hair was tied back in a black bandana, exposing an earlobe that had been shorn into three parts by earrings that had torn through her flesh.

"I like you to examine my baby," she said, shifting in her chair and pulling Ezekiel up by his shoulder higher onto her lap. She turned the baby to face me. "See, he don't look so good. What you think's wrong with him?"

He was a scrawny little thing, much too small for five months, sitting, somewhat limply, on his mother's lap. Snot dripped from his nose and drool was flowing over his chin, dripping onto his T-shirt. He kept looking up and reaching for his mother's face.

I proceeded to get some basic medical history. Ezekiel was born of a normal pregnancy with no complications. He did well in the newborn period and went home with his mother two days after birth. There was no history of any diseases, such as sickle cell disease or diabetes, that ran in the family. His medical history was basically uncomplicated, and gave no indication of why he should not be growing properly.

"Who lives at home with you and Ezekiel?" I asked his mom.

"There's me, and the other ones. I got two living with me now. The city took the others away. They said I wasn't taking care of them. They don't know what they is talking about. I'm going to try and get them back." She became visibly upset, shook her head and looked down at the ground. "I love my children. I don't like nobody taking them away from me."

"Is there anyone else in the house?" I asked. Through all this Ezekiel sat in his mother's lap, propped between her breast and her arm, playing with a tassel hanging off her dress.

"Naw. Just them and my girlfriend and her two kids."

"Is Ezekiel's father involved?"

"Yeah, he comes and visits me every day. We care about each other, you know what I mean? He comes by every day and helps out with the kids."

I looked down at Ezekiel sitting in his mother's lap. She said she loved him, so why had she waited four months to bring him into the office when he wasn't growing? We all mean different things when we refer to love, and some of us are fortunate enough to be able to translate our loving feelings into deeds. She must have been overwhelmed by the need to care for yet another child. At twenty-three, most of the people I grew up with were in graduate schools cramming for exams, not struggling to keep their lives together in streets filled with cocaine while bringing up their sixth child.

I tried to see if Ezekiel would focus on my eyes. He was slow to focus at first, but then our eyes connected and he smiled back as I made faces at him. I shined a small penlight onto one of his fingers. He seemed interested in the light, as a child his age was supposed to be, and tried to pull the penlight to his mouth. I would hold the penlight in front of him and he would reach for it, though he seemed to need more encouragement than most kids his age would need.

I asked his mother to put him down on the examination table. Lying still on the table he looked like a young bird fallen from its nest, his rib cage rising with each thin breath, skin clinging to each rib. He turned toward me as I scratched the tabletop, then he reached his hand toward my finger. His small hand wrapped around my forefinger with a solid grip, and he held onto my finger as I moved it over his chest to the other side of his body. Both of our heads tilted as we looked at our fingers in the air.

"What do you think is wrong with him?" his mother's voice jolted me. She was impatient and nervous.

"Let me examine him," I replied in a tight voice. It disturbs me when someone allows a problem to fester for months and then demands an immediate answer.

I started from the top of his body. The soft spot on his head felt normal. His eyes followed me around the room. His heart sounded clear and strong with no abnormal murmurs, his liver felt normal in size. Other than a terrible diaper rash everything looked and felt normal. Except Ezekiel looked terrible and washed out, with eyes sunken, skin stretched over his bones, and a blank expression on his face.

I asked his mom more questions: What was he eating? How often did he eat? How much water did she give him between feedings? How much time did she spend playing with him each day? Where did he sleep? In a crib, on a cot, or in bed with her? What was her day like? What did she do during the day? How did she feel about taking care of

Ezekiel along with all the other responsibilities that she had to deal with?

She answered all the questions. He was getting a sufficient amount of an iron-containing formula. She found things to be a lot of work, but she loved her child and that was work she had to do. I excused myself from the room and sat down in my office. If she was doing all the proper things, why did he look so bad? I tried to sort out the different possibilities and what I could do about them. Most probably, Ezekiel was not growing because he just wasn't receiving enough food and attention. Many medical studies over the last twenty years have shown this to be the most common cause of an infant's failure to thrive, especially if there are no physical abnormalities pointing to disease. It is hard, though, to be sure of this diagnosis through the history obtained from the child's parent.

I sat in my office thinking. Ezekiel was in the examination room lying on the table. If I felt he was in danger over the next few days—the law uses the term *imminent danger*—I could file a petition with the city's child welfare division and admit Ezekiel to the hospital this afternoon. During his hospital stay the people from the Department of Human Services could assess Ezekiel's home environment while we were keeping a careful eye on him. If he gained weight as he was fed and cuddled in the hospital, it would suggest that his failure to thrive was due to social problems that prevented him from receiving the food and attention he needed.

The benefits of admitting him to the hospital were simple and straightforward. The risks, particularly with regard to his family, were not. Taking Ezekiel away from his mother was likely to undermine her confidence in her ability to take care of Ezekiel and her other children. It would also interfere with the development of a trusting doctor-patient relationship between his mother and me, a relationship that would take on greater importance during Ezekiel's continuing care. If I felt that Ezekiel was not in imminent danger, the best choice might be to somehow work with Ezekiel's mother, to get her to pay more attention to Ezekiel despite everything else that was going on in her life.

I decided that I would draw a set of blood tests to check for any medical illness that might be causing his failure to thrive, and see Ezekiel back in the office in one week. While waiting for the blood-test results to come back from the lab, I would also get the city's social workers to make an assessment of Ezekiel's home environment.

Walking down the hall to Ezekiel's examination room, I wondered if I was doing the right thing. What if something happened to Ezekiel over the next week? I wondered if it mattered at all what I decided. Would any intervention that I could recommend affect how Ezekiel turned out by the time he was twenty years old? I knew the odds were stacked strongly against Ezekiel and that it was unlikely that he would grow up to be a policeman, doctor, or lawyer—and not because he did not have the potential. It was because, despite whatever efforts I could make, he would go back to an environment where the expression of love is often stunted, or ends up being traded as a commodity on a street corner for a line of cocaine.

I walked into the room where Ezekiel's mother sat, playing with Ezekiel on her lap. She looked up and said,

"Well, what you think's wrong with him? What you think he needs? Vitamins?"

"I think we need to do some blood tests," I said. "We need to check to see how his kidneys are working, and his liver. That will mean drawing blood."

I explained to her that I could tell that she was a caring mother and that she was trying hard. I suggested to her that while we were waiting for the blood-test results she should try especially hard to pay attention to Ezekiel and make an effort to feed him every four hours. I also told her that a child welfare worker would be out to see her in a few days, and that I wanted to see her back in the office in a week. She looked tired and nodded quietly as she got Ezekial dressed.

During the next week a social worker visited their apartment. The social worker told me over the phone that Ezekiel and his mother were living, along with Ezekiel's brother and sister and another family, in an old, run-down apartment building with no running water or electricity. To get the tap water that had to be added to Ezekiel's concentrated infant formula, his mother had to walk a block and a half to her mother's apartment and carry the water back in a plastic jar. Also, because the gas for the stove had been shut off, there was no way for her to warm the baby's milk. The social worker had contacted the water and the gas companies to turn the utilities back on.

Ezekiel and his mother showed up right on time for their next appointment. When I walked into the examination room Ezekiel was again lying across his mother's lap. She was wearing the same black-and-red striped dress; his head was dangling over her thigh. This time his mother looked a little more nervous, more on edge, than she had before. She had also brought her other two children and Ezekiel's father with her. The room smelled of urine that came from the two-year-old, who was now playing with a handle that he had unscrewed from the bottom drawer of the examination table. Ezekiel's father was a big, muscular man who towered over me as we shook hands. He had a powerful grip and thick calluses on his fingers. His forearm was as thick as a tree limb and I noticed track marks running along its side.

"I want to thank you for taking such good care of Ezekiel," he said in a deep voice. "There're not a lot a people interested in seeing how a child's doing. I been there. I been on drugs and now I'm clean, and I'm gonna stay clean. I want something better for my child. I know you're going to help him. I got real confidence in you."

Confidence in me. It was disturbing to have such confidence placed in me, when I knew how little I had to offer, or rather, how little I had to offer compared to what they had to offer themselves, if only they could tap into it.

One of my functions, I have come to realize, is to lead people, or trick them, into helping themselves. It is like a magician's illusion. Someone comes in with a headache they've had for a week. I examine them and tell them there is nothing serious causing their headache. Then the headache goes away the next day. If I gave them a pill they would think that I "cured" their headache. In fact, I have done nothing but tell them they are fine; they cured the headache on their own.

The same thing often happens, hopefully happens, with

children who are not growing because of social problems at home. The social problems have distracted the mother's attention from the infant. When I refocus the mother's attention back on her child, when I ask her to record the hours the child eats and how much he eats, the child starts to gain weight again. I have seen this happen a number of times. The cure resides within the patient and the patient's family. With luck the doctor can sometimes help the family realize its potential.

"Zeke's looking better since you seen him last week. He's doing better already," the father said, and smiled at me. He was missing one of his front teeth, and the one next to it was rotting.

Ezekiel was sitting up playing with a tassel of his mother's dress. She kept fidgeting around in her chair, combing her fingers through his hair, sitting him up straighter in her lap, then back down again, pulling his diapers up a bit, then readjusting them back down to where they were. We discussed his diet over the last week. He was eating the "same as usual," she said, six ounces of formula every four or five hours. I picked Ezekiel up and placed him on the scale. Twelve ounces heavier than the week before. I examined him. Nothing new on his physical examination. His diaper rash still looked bad, but it was improving.

I heard something crash on the floor. I turned around and found that the two-year-old had climbed up on the chair, knocked over a jar of sterile swabs, and was putting a handful of them in his mouth. His mother slapped him. "I told you not to touch nothing, now sit down," she snapped. Then to me, "He's always getting into things."

I helped her pick up the swabs. The three-year-old had

picked some up and started throwing them at his brother. "Stop that now or I'm going to whip you," she yelled and slapped at his arm. They had been in the office less than ten minutes, my floor looked like a large game of pick-up sticks, and I was beginning to feel outnumbered. Dealing with the energy of these two kids was what her life consisted of all day long, and at the same time she had to care for Ezekiel. She had to do all this in an apartment where there had been no running water and no working stove. I couldn't imagine being able to handle that, and yet she had to, or I and the Department of Human Services could take away her youngest child.

I explained to her that Ezekiel's blood tests had all come back normal. His kidneys, liver, and thyroid were all working well. The main reason he was not gaining weight, I told her, was that he appeared to be the type of child that needs a lot of attention, and needs his feedings at regular intervals during the day. If he was not given that extra attention then he would not gain weight. Just with the increased attention that she and the baby's father had been paying him over the last week he had gained a good deal of weight and was back on the right track. I complimented them on their ability to provide Ezekiel the attention that he needed. I explained how important it was for them to focus on Ezekiel and his feedings. All this time Ezekiel was lying on his belly on the examination table playing with a swab that had landed next to him.

"It's hard . . ." Ezekiel's mother began, looking as if she were about to cry. Then she gulped, sat up straight, and with a proud look said, "I love my baby. I'd do anything for my baby. If you say pay attention to him, I'll pay attention to him. I want to do what's good for my baby."

I looked at the two-year-old with his wet pants, crouched in the corner, looking up out of the sides of his eyes. Ezekiel's father was standing by the door holding the three-year-old's hand.

"Let me ask you something," she said, and then hesitated. "I been feeling nauseous. Would you be my doctor? I need a good doctor."

"What's wrong?"

"I'm feeling nauseous, and my stomach feels bad. Down here at the bottom," she pointed to her pelvis.

I handed her an examination gown and left the room so she could change. Many things can cause nausea and pelvic discomfort. Unfortunately, one thing was most likely.

I came back into the room with the nurse. Ezekiel's mother was sitting on the examination table. The children and Ezekiel's father were out in the waiting room. I asked her to lie down and show me where she was uncomfortable. She pointed at the loose folds of skin beneath her navel. I examined her belly, and she did not seem tender. Then I put on my gloves and performed a pelvic examination. As much as I was prepared for it, I had trouble believing my own hands.

I told her, "It looks like you're about twelve weeks pregnant."

A Soft Snow Falling

SONETA FIRST WALKED into my office on a snowy January afternoon, bundled in a red wool sweater, a wool cap, and a long gray overcoat. It had been snowing most of the previous night and morning, and I was surprised to see her, since the weather had kept most of our other patients from showing up for their appointments. I picked up her chart and read the nurse's note. Soneta had come in because for two months she had a nagging cough, lack of energy, and weight loss. She also had a temperature of 103°.

When I walked into the examination room I found Soneta sitting hunched over on the examination table, holding the edge for support with both hands. Her cheeks were sunken and her large bloodshot eyes stared straight toward the floor. Her thin legs dangled from the table. Her hair was thin and bunched up on the back of her head. She looked more like a woman of eighty than one of twenty-three. I introduced myself, then asked her to explain to me how she had been feeling.

"I don't know," she said, still staring at the floor. She seemed uncomfortably shy. "I been with this cough a month or two now. Been feeling tired. Lousy. Like I don't got no energy. And I lost some weight. I don't know. I wasn't gonna come in, but I figured I'd get checked out."

I asked her about other symptoms and there really weren't any. Then I performed her physical exam. Eyes, nose, throat, lungs. Everything looked normal. In fact, the thing most remarkable about her exam was how comfortable she looked for a woman who was running a fever of 103°. And how thin she appeared. She was shrunken. Her wrists looked like young birch sprouts, the muscles of her neck stood out like taut rope, and her thin skin hugged the crevice of her collarbone. I explained to her that I thought we should check some blood samples and a chest x-ray and asked her to come back to see me in the office in two days. I walked out of the exam room and down the hall. Looking out the window I watched soft snowflakes covering the street, sidewalk, and parked cars. A block away the housing projects loomed over the neighborhood like a snow-covered mountain over the surrounding valley.

Soneta's tests results came back the next day. Her sedimentation rate, an indicator of serious disease, and her white blood count, a sign of infection, were both elevated. More important was her chest x-ray, which revealed a white lacy pattern over the upper lobes of her lungs, classic for tuberculosis.

When Soneta came back the next day for her follow-up appointment, she was wearing the same red wool sweater and gray overcoat. "All of the lab results have come back," I told her. "It appears that what has been causing your cough, weight loss, and fever is tuberculosis."

Soneta did not say a thing. She continued to stare straight ahead with bloodshot eyes.

"Tuberculosis is a type of bacteria, a germ," I went on, "that infects the lungs. It is a serious infection, as you know by the way you have been feeling." Soneta's eyes were now avoiding mine, and she began curling her lower lip between her teeth. She did not say a thing as I explained to her the details of her disease. Once in the lungs, TB causes a slowly progressive, often devastating pneumonia. Before modern drug therapy, individuals infected with tuberculosis spent years wasting away, which is why the disease had been called "consumption." Fortunately, tuberculosis is fully treatable with modern medicines. I spent about forty-five minutes with Soneta. I told her we would check samples of the sputum she was coughing up. Then I explained to her about the antituberculosis medications—that they would have to be taken every day, that she would need to be on medication for a full six months, that I would have to see her monthly to make sure she was not having any adverse reactions. I recommended that she get her boy-friend and her daughter tested for TB since they might have been exposed. I also explained that one of the medica-tions would make her urine turn orange, and that she wasn't to worry, because this was a normal side effect.

Throughout our conversation Soneta stared at the floor, shifting weight in her seat. When I asked her if what I was saying made sense, she told me it did. When I asked her to repeat to me what I'd just told her, she was able to do so easily, though in a dreary monotone.

I wrote out the prescriptions for her medications, and told her that I would like to see her back in the office in a week. Staring at the floor, she took the prescriptions, mum-bled thanks, and walked out the door.

When Soneta returned to the office a week later she seemed brighter and more talkative than she had the week before. Perhaps the medications were taking effect; perhaps she was just in a better mood.

"You look better this week than last," I told her, smiling.

"Yeah," she said shyly. "I'm feeling a little better."

"Have you had any problems taking the medicines?"

"Nope, no problems. My boyfriend and my daughter went and got checked like you said, and they're OK."

"Good. As long as you are doing well, let me see you back in the office in three weeks." I felt satisfied that I had made her diagnosis and that she was now on the appropriate medications.

Over the next three months Soneta missed a number of appointments. After each missed appointment, she would call, apologize to the receptionist, and schedule another office visit. She did not come back to the office until late March, the first week of spring. When I walked in, Soneta was sitting in a small chair next to the examination table. She looked as though she had lost ten pounds from her tiny frame. Her cheekbones jutted from her face, creating dark sockets in which her bloodshot eyes nervously darted back and forth, like a figure from an Edvard Munch painting. Her red linen shirt hung off the bones of her shoulders as if it were hanging from a clothes hanger, with no body beneath it.

"Where have you been?" I blurted out, shocked by the way she looked.

She stared over my left shoulder for a second, then began shaking her head. "I don't know. . . . I . . . I'm not getting any better. I been meaning to come in, but . . . you know . . . things just keep getting in the way. I take my medicine every day, but I ain't getting no better."

"Are you still having fevers?"

"Every night. And I'm coughing ugly yellow stuff up. I'm coughing all night. I can't stop coughing," she replied.

I pulled out my stethoscope, placed it against the back of her chest, and listened carefully. With each deep breath, her lungs sounded like an ocean wave breaking against a cliff. I shook my head and stepped back.

"Your lungs don't sound good. We will need to send off some blood and sputum samples and repeat a chest x-ray to figure out what is going on. I'd like you to come back here in two days to go over the results."

That afternoon I received a call from the hospital radiologist. He told me that Soneta's chest x-ray had thick white infiltrates of disease throughout the upper and middle lobes of her lungs. It looked a great deal worse than the x-ray from three months before. He had not seen a chest x-ray like Soneta's in thirty years, he told me, since he had first begun his medical practice with the public health service in a small rural town in south Georgia. The chest x-ray looked like advanced, untreated tuberculosis.

I hung up the phone, leaned back in my chair, and looked out the window. It was raining outside and the boarded-up brick building across the street glistened with a thin coat of water. It was unclear to me why Soneta was not getting better. The cultures that we took of her sputum showed that her tuberculosis should have been cured by the medicines I had prescribed for her; nonetheless, if she continued to get worse she might die. I watched two children dressed in yellow raincoats and boots splash at each other across a puddle on the sidewalk in front of the abandoned building. I picked up the phone and dialed Soneta's number. She would need to be admitted to the hospital for intravenous antibiotic therapy. When she answered I asked her to pack her suitcase and go down to the admissions department of the hospital. For a long stay.

A medical student met Soneta in the emergency room and performed the first of the five physical exams that Soneta would have that day. Soneta had patience with the student and talked to her at length. Then I examined her. By the time the third-year resident examined Soneta, and then the infectious-disease fellow, and then the infectious-disease consultant, all asking if she had taken her medicines, all asking if she was *sure* that she was taking her medicines, all asking her if she had used intravenous drugs or if she had ever been a prostitute, Soneta decided that she was going to stop talking to people and just sat in her bed staring out the window and biting her lip. By the end of the day she was labeled as uncooperative by the consultants and the house-staff physicians.

At the end of the afternoon I stopped back in Soneta's room to see how she was doing. Outside her door, in accordance with hospital regulations, I pulled a surgical mask from its cardboard box and placed it over my face, to decrease the chance of contracting tuberculosis and spreading it to other patients. When I walked in the room my eyes were drawn to a large picture window opposite the door. Through the window swaying branches of a bare tree were silhouetted by lights in large office buildings and an orange-maroon sky. The tree was growing in a square of dirt carved from the concrete sidewalk below. Soneta was sitting in her bed angrily staring at me.

"What you have to admit me to the hospital for?" she snapped, her head lurching forward. "What all these people asking me the same dumb questions for? Got to come in and bother me when I ain't feeling good? Why don't they ask each other?"

I looked at her. She was sitting in bed, with the hospital gown hanging like loose skin below her head, eyes bulging out, swaying back and forth like a cobra, full of venom. Although I didn't make her sick, I was the one who had told her she was ill. I was the one who essentially gave her disease to her. Before she came to see me she was a healthy young woman who had weight loss and a cough. After she left my office, she had tuberculosis. I was the one who had told her to come into the hospital, and because of whom she was now being put through the indignities of multiple people walking into her room, asking her if she was a whore, and then examining her body. It would have been understandable if she hated me, but she also needed me. I was her only link within the hospital to the person she had been on the outside, before she was ill. I had seen her, if only for a few minutes, before she ever had tuberculosis, or knew that she had it, before she had lost additional weight to become the near corpse she now was. She also knew that I controlled, to some extent, what would happen to her during her hospital stay, what drugs she would get, what tests would be performed, and what doctors would be called in to see her. Her relationship with me was a tangle of hate and need.

I didn't know how to respond to her questions. She was right. It was insulting and inconsiderate to have five people examine her, yet that is how the system works. Often it works for the good of the patient. Sometimes one person finds out information in the history that no one else has, or thinks of a diagnostic test or a medication while talking to the patient that no one else has thought of. Seeing the patient, examining the patient with your own hands and eyes, getting a *sense* for the patient and the disease process that may be going on, is quite different than cogitating over the story of the patient as conveyed to you by another physician, and that sense of the patient can open up different and productive channels of thought. Nonetheless, it is intimidating and bothersome to patients when many people examine them on admission to the hospital, when they are feeling their worst. Especially when the examination is not done, as can happen, with the utmost consideration and respect.

I didn't know what to say to her, so I told her what most doctors tell their patients at times like this—that I was sorry she had to go through all of this, that I know she didn't like it, but that it was important for her and was for her own good. Then I said good night, because I was hungry, and left her to stew in her own thoughts.

The next morning the hospital team, which was composed of two medical students, two interns, a resident, and myself, were making our daily rounds when the intern was paged to the nurse's station. He needed to come right away, the nurse told him, because Soneta was yelling and threatening to leave the hospital unless she could talk to a doctor immediately. We all went to her room together to see what the problem was.

The six of us walked down the hall, stopped to put on surgical masks, and filed into Soneta's room. She was sitting straight up on the side of her bed, swaying back and forth in jerky motions. She was tapping on her legs with both her hands and chewing on her twitching lower lip. Her hospital gown was hanging off of one shoulder, barely covering her chest, and her head moved back and forth as she watched each one of us as we walked through the door. Then she focused on me.

"What are you doing to me here?" she demanded. "I went to the bathroom and peed out orange. Why's my body doing that? What's that from?"

"Well, that's because . . ." and I stopped. Rifampin, one of the antituberculosis drugs that I had prescribed for her three months ago, tints all body secretions with an orange hue. If she had been taking rifampin for three months, the orange color of her urine would not have been new to her. As it was, she was terrified. She must not have had orange urine before, which meant that she had not been taking her medications. This explained why her tuberculosis had progressed to an advanced stage.

I looked toward the third-year resident, who was not really listening and was standing, tired and bored, looking out the window. I glanced at the medical student, who was watching carefully, and nodded.

"Were you taking the medicines at home?" I asked Soneta.

"Yeah. I told you I did," she replied, staring straight at me. Her eyes darted up and to the side, then back toward me.

"Were you really?"

"I was taking my pills," she said. "You asked me and I already told you."

I hesitated to ask her more questions—it seemed so unfair, with all of us in the room. But I needed to know, and later the opportunity to find out might be lost.

"How often were you missing your pills?" I asked.

She paused.

"Sometimes I miss one," she said.

She looked over toward the corner of the room where no one was standing. There was an uncomfortable silence. She shifted position and pulled her gown back up onto her shoulders.

"The orange color of your urine," I explained, "is a normal reaction to one of the antituberculosis medicines that you are taking. If you had been taking the medicines all along you would have been used to the orange color of your urine."

I paused for a moment. She began shaking. I continued, "How often did you really miss taking the medicines? It's important for us to know in order to know what medications to give you now."

"Well . . ." she hesitated, then turned back toward me, slumped over. She was looking down into her lap. She picked up a blanket lying by her leg and held it in her lap.

"Yes?"

Her eyes were riveted on the blanket as she began rolling the edge between her fingers. Her voice started to crack as she began, "I guess . . . I . . . I guess . . . pretty often . . . I just . . . I think . . ."

She shifted uncomfortably in the thin hospital gown

that had no back and that barely covered her body to her mid-thigh. The six of us in our starched white coats stood still as ice in her room.

"I know," she said, and began to sob. "I know."

Over the next four weeks we gave Soneta strong intravenous and oral antibiotics; nonetheless, she grew steadily weaker and lost more weight. Each night she ran fevers of 102° to 104°, drenching her sheets with sweat. Once a week we repeated her chest x-ray. Once a week we would stand in the radiology viewing room and interpret her x-ray as having larger areas of white, diseased lung where healthy, dark areas should have been. Our medications were having little effect.

Each morning Soneta coughed up large globs of yellow phlegm that had collected in her lungs while she slept. During paroxysms of coughing her bed would shake. Afterward she would have trouble catching her breath. On Monday mornings, during rounds, we would hand Soneta a sterile plastic container and ask her to collect a sample of phlegm to send to the lab.

Monday afternoons, the members of our team would gather in the microbiology lab where the sputum sample had been stained to make the tubercular organisms appear bright red under the microscope. We would look to see if there was any decrease in the number of tuberculosis bacilli Soneta was coughing up. Taking turns peering into the eyepiece of the microscope, we would see abundant, glowing red slashes spread over a purple background, like red commas scattered across a written page. We could also see round, light purple leukocytes, the body's main defense against disease, with their darker blue, many-lobed nuclei. Sometimes we would see a tuberculosis bacillus engulfed by a leukocyte. Viewed at a magnification of one thousand, the stained sample of her sputum looked like a beautiful red-and-purple fresco, a microscopic world frozen in a dance of death.

The course of Soneta's illness was as perplexing as it was disturbing. Neither the infectious-disease consultants nor I had ever seen a case of TB this resistant to treatment in an otherwise young, healthy woman. Was there a reason the antibiotics seemed unable to fight off the bacteria? We searched for signs of other illnesses that might have impaired her immune system—AIDS or lymphoma—but these tests were negative. I believe the course of Soneta's illness sent all the doctors caring for her to the library and to phone consultations with tuberculosis specialists to see if we could find anything we were not thinking of that might help her.

I began my own literature search in the usual places: textbooks of infectious diseases, textbooks of antimicrobial therapy, recent articles on tuberculosis. Most of these sources, though, discussed the treatment of TB in patients who began treatment shortly after acquiring the disease. Few of the articles specifically addressed untreated tuberculosis, which was essentially what Soneta had for the first three months of her illness, when she was not taking her medications. I began to look up older articles, published in the 1940s when antibiotics were first being introduced for the treatment of TB. I examined the course of the disease in the placebo and the experimental groups, and I noticed that the progress of Soneta's illness mimicked the course of the illness in individuals with severe disease in the placebo groups.

As I read the older articles, I became more aware of the ravages of tuberculosis before antibiotics were available. Tuberculosis is transmitted through small droplets that are suspended in the air when a person who has tuberculosis coughs. When another individual in close proximity breathes in these droplets, that person can contract the disease. This is why tuberculosis is more common in individuals who live in crowded conditions. As the Industrial Revolution drew people into the cities during the late 1700s and 1800s, tuberculosis became the most common identifiable cause of death. More than one-fourth of all adult deaths in Europe during the eighteenth and nineteenth centuries were caused by tuberculosis. Not surprisingly, the effects of tuberculosis permeated the culture of the era. Among those afflicted were authors, musicians, and artists; they included Henry David Thoreau, Emily Brontë, John Keats, Robert Louis Stevenson, Frédéric Chopin, and Franz Kafka.

It is only in the past forty years that antibiotics have become a part of our ordinary armamentarium against disease. Streptomycin, the first effective antituberculosis medication, first became available in 1944. Prior to that time, tuberculosis patients were sent to sanitariums deep in the countryside or high in the mountains, in the hopes that the sun and fresh air would help their natural defenses fight off the disease. If the climate didn't help, at least they would be out of the crowded city and so would not spread the disease to others.

Effective antibiotics have decreased the threat of tuberculosis for most people living in civilized countries today. In the United States, tuberculosis is so rare now that most doctors do not see even one case a year. The low rates of tuberculosis across the country, however, do not reflect the situation in many inner-city neighborhoods, where the incidence of tuberculosis is up to twenty times that in middle-class communities. Crowded living conditions, poor nutrition, and less access to quality medical care all contribute to increased rates of tuberculosis.

The library search, although it helped to put Soneta's plight in historical perspective, did not uncover any new information to help arrest the course of Soneta's disease. Our infectious-disease consultant made several long-distance calls to one of the world's experts on tuberculosis at the Jewish Hospital in Denver, to ask for any suggestions he might have. His recommendation was that we increase our antibiotic coverage from four to six different strong medications.

After six weeks in the hospital, Soneta was no longer getting up to sit in the chair by her bed. She spent her days lying on her side in a fetal position, with a bed sheet pulled over her head. She seemed to be slowly sinking into her mattress, like a lost traveler disappearing into quicksand.

Next to her bed, on her night table, she kept a pitcher of water and a box of tissues. The curtains in her room were drawn, and the overhead lights were always off. At mid-day the darkness of her room was broken only by a beam of sunlight that entered through a small space between the curtains. Just visible through that space, the budding branches of a white magnolia tree swayed in the breeze, almost touching the window.

Soneta's mother and twelve-year-old daughter visited her every day, usually at about four in the afternoon. Before walking into Soneta's room they would put on green surgical masks. The masks reached from below their chins, over their cheeks and noses, to just below their eyes. Their visits would usually last about two hours. Each day on their way out of the hospital they would find Soneta's nurse and ask her why Soneta wasn't looking better yet, and when she would be coming home. The nurse would explain that the treatment for tuberculosis took a long time and that things were still unpredictable. This became a ritual that they repeated every day.

During the rare times when Soneta was allowed to leave her room, usually to get a chest x-ray, hospital rules required that she wear a mask to protect other patients from contracting tuberculosis. In every conversation that Soneta had during the six weeks that she had been in the hospital, either she or the person she was talking to was wearing a mask; it had been six weeks since Soneta communicated face to face with another human being. When Soneta's daughter smiled as she walked in the room, Soneta could not see her smile. When her daughter felt like crying, as she must have at times, sitting with her mother caged in that room, Soneta might not have known it until her daughter's eyes became restless and flooded with tears.

I handed a request card to the radiology file clerk and buttoned my white coat for warmth. The hospital had just turned on its air conditioners for the summer. The clerk pulled out a manila folder containing Soneta's chest x-rays. I took the films, walked past the other members of the team to the viewing box, and flicked on the light switch. I placed the current x-ray in front of me, positioned the x-ray from two weeks before to its left, and looked at the intern.

"Her tuberculosis is still progressing," the intern said with a stern look, comparing the two films. The resident and two medical students nodded in agreement. The intern continued, "Her infiltrate is much denser bilaterally, and she has fluid in the left base of her lung." He shook his head. "Is it true that she didn't take her medicines for three months before coming into the hospital?"

Since students and residents rotated to different services in the hospital every four weeks, this was the third group that I had worked with while taking care of Soneta. Each group was more distant from the circumstances surrounding her admission than was the group before. When this present hospital team met Soneta, she was already a frail, depressed woman who never got out of bed.

"Yes, that's what happened," I responded dully. I wasn't in a mood for discussing more details.

"That's too bad," the intern replied, shaking his head. "You can't help those people. Thanks for going over the x-rays with us. We're going to go and finish afternoon rounds, then we'll all sign out about four-thirty, OK?"

"OK," I said, and turned back to look at the x-ray again as the team left the room.

Soneta's chest x-ray was filled more densely than before with thick white infiltrates of disease. It was as though swirling storm clouds had dumped a thick layer of snow over the whole film. Her bronchial tree, seen through the white haze that covered the upper portion of her lungs, looked like branches barely visible in the distance of a snow storm. A white drift of disease rode up against her heart on the left side of her lung like a snowbank leaning against a house. Scattered white patches, like storm clouds, covered large portions of both lungs. The progression, when compared with the x-ray from two weeks earlier, was striking.

I thought back six months to that snowy January afternoon when I first met Soneta, when she was huddled in a thin sweater and an overcoat. I remembered her telling me about her cough, and how shocked I was when she took off her sweater and I saw how thin she was. It seemed like so long ago. I turned around to see if anyone else was standing in the viewing room. There was no one else there, and I was thankful for this. In the hospital, it is a rare but needed luxury to have the solitude to gather one's thoughts.

I looked back at the x-ray and took a deep breath. This young woman was continuing to deteriorate every week and there was nothing more I or anyone else could do for her. I was angry, frustrated, and upset. What about Soneta so upset me? Why couldn't I just blame her, as the intern had, so I would not have to feel for her? I know how easy it is to shield oneself from the pain of tragedies that occur to strangers. I had known Soneta for six months, and though I did not feel as if I knew her well, I believe there must have been a reason, a sad reason, for the quiet distance she put up between herself and her doctors. Soneta was three years younger than I was, and she was dying.

Three physicians walked through the door to the viewing room, talking with each other and smiling. I nodded hello, took the chest films down from the viewing box, and returned them to the file clerk. Then I walked out the door and down the hallway to Soneta's room.

Outside the door I took a surgical mask from the cardboard box, pulled the straps over my ears, and positioned it on my face. When I walked in Soneta was lying on her side, her head propped up by three pillows, a white sheet covering her body to mid-chest. The room was dim, and through the crack in the curtains I could see the brilliant white blossoms of the magnolia tree caressing the window. A ray of sunlight streamed in, traveled across the room, and landed in a blaze on the gray wall above the head of Soneta's bed.

Soneta looked toward me. An intravenous line entered the skin below her collar bone, dripping yellow fluid into her body. Beads of sweat were dripping from her forehead, and her chest was heaving rapidly. She looked like a worn-out mountain climber who had collapsed at an altitude where the air is too thin to breathe. Then her eyes turned away, toward the white ceiling, looking as if she were indeed a mountain climber, too weak now to overcome one more obstacle; who, seeing the sun setting behind the distant summit, its yellow light scattering in rainbows through crystal rivulets of ice, stares out at the terrible beauty of a soft snow beginning to fall.

A Stitch in Time

I WALK INTO the small exam room and Lucretia is sitting in the corner, her arms folded across her chest and her ankles crossed underneath her chair. She is looking down at the ground. I hold out my hand and say hello. She looks up briefly, then, looking back down, she begins, "The doctor in the emergency room put fifteen stitches in. He told me to get them out in about a week. I been trying to come in but I been real busy." Then she hands me the instruction sheet from the emergency room and points to the right side of her head. "It's time I get them out."

"OK," I reply, and glance at the sheet. The stitches were placed in early February, almost a month ago. I walk over to her and position the examination lamp over the side of her head. Fifteen crisscrossed stitches form a line across the right side of her scalp. Around each stitch is a crust of dried blood. I pull a plastic glove over my hand and run my fingers over the wound, feeling the prickly ends of the sutures sticking through her skin. As a physician—touching lacerations, palpating abdomens, pressing armpits for swollen glands—I often feel like a blind man reading braille, searching with my fingertips for encoded bits of information that will tell me something of worlds I cannot see. There is no evidence of infection below the wound and the wound itself is neither tender nor warm. I pick up the suture removal kit from the examination table.

Lucretia shifts in her seat and looks around me toward the door. "Will this take long?" she mutters, rubbing her forehead.

"Just a few minutes. Now turn your head to the side, keep still, and I'll take the stitches out." Removing her sutures will be a nice break in an otherwise hectic day, a simple, straightforward procedure that should take about five minutes. When I'm done I'll be ahead of schedule and I'll be able to feel a little more comfortable taking my time with the sick child in the next room.

I reposition the examination lamp over her laceration, then grasp the nylon suture nearest her ear with the forceps and gently lift her skin up as I pull on the thread. "How did you cut yourself?" I ask, slipping the scissors under the stitch and snipping the first suture.

"An accident."

I put the crusted suture in the bottom of the empty suture removal kit. Later, if I lose count, I can check the number of sutures I have removed. Her head is turned toward the ground, away from the light. I grasp the second suture with my forceps.

"What kind of accident?" I slip the scissors under the second stitch, snip it, and pull the thread from her skin.

"You know, an accident," she replies, shaking her head. She sounds irritated as she says the word *accident*.

"Please don't move your head," I tell her, and reposition the lamp again so the focus of the light falls back on her stitches. I wipe some crust from over the third suture.

She begins wringing her hands together. It is clear that she does not want to talk. I try to judge where the boundary lies between providing good medical care and invading her privacy. I step back and I ask again, "What kind of accident?"

She looks up and stares straight into my eyes. The bright examination lamp is shining from behind her to her right, lighting up her laceration and casting a shadow over the left side of her face.

"I got jumped," she says, holding my eyes for a second, then looking back down at the floor.

"Do you know who jumped you?" I ask.

"Yeah. . . ." Her voice is quivering. "A friend." She twists her body toward the far wall, stares at the sink, and begins shaking her head. Her legs are crossed at the ankle and tucked tightly under her chair. In the background I hear the faint cry of an infant in an exam room down the hall.

"A friend?" I ask, and pause. She is staring silently at the floor. "Who was it?"

She begins kneading her hands together again. Her eyes are closed. She takes two deep breaths.

"My man," she says. She opens her eyes for a moment to look at me, then closes them and drops her head into her hands. "That's who."

I feel her embarrassment and her shame. I question whether I should have pushed her as I did; she came in only to get her sutures taken out. Yet perhaps I can help her in a way she could not have anticipated. Perhaps I can encourage her to get help.

"That must be awful," I reply, not knowing what to say. I hesitate, then continue. "Is this the same man you've been with for a while?" Before walking into the examination room I glanced at her chart and noticed that three months ago she had been treated for gonorrhea. I remember now that at the time, she believed she had gotten the infection from a man she was living with.

"Yeah, two and a half years."

I put the forceps and scissors back on the examination table and sit back down in my chair. "Has he ever hit you before?" I ask.

"No. This was the first time," she says, still staring at the floor.

"Are you sure?"

"Yes. . . ." She hesitates again. She begins shaking her head and continues, her voice now a higher pitch. "No. It wasn't the first time, but it was never this bad before. This is the first time I needed stitches."

"What happened?"

"He just came in from outside and started yelling. Maybe he was smoking crack, maybe he was drinking. He was pissed off about something. Then he started pushing me. Asking me why wasn't his dinner ready yet. The he starts saying why was I such a whore, was I out whoring or something with my friends, was that why dinner wasn't ready. And I says no, I just got in from work, but he says, 'Work, bullshit. You was out whoring. You was out sucking men,' and then he tells me, 'You my woman.' And then he turns around, and says, 'I'll teach you,' and he shoves me up against the wall. And I says stop it and he shoves me down on the couch and he is cursing at me and picks up the lamp on the table and slams me upside my head. The lamp broke into pieces and I was bleeding, and my son was crying and hitting him and telling him to get away."

I listen as Lucretia pours out her story. As she talks she wrings her hands and her whole body begins shaking. As she continues to talk the shaking becomes less, she grows calmer. She needed to tell someone what happened. She needs someone to listen to her.

I sit, able only to listen. A few minutes earlier, I had walked into her exam room intending to remove fifteen sutures. I asked a few questions and then Lucretia started talking about what was really going on. When I think of the pain that Lucretia is living with, I also think of the hidden pains so many of my patients have that I am unaware of because I don't ask the right questions. Failing to ask the right questions, I spend my time treating superficial manifestations of underlying problems that I don't even know exist—as when I treated Lucretia for bruises six months ago and today almost took out her sutures without suspecting that her main problem was that she was being physically abused by her boyfriend.

Lucretia continues, "I grabbed my son and ran out of the house. My head was bleeding so I ripped off the end of my shirt and held it where he hit me. Then I went to the emergency room and they put in fifteen stitches."

"It sounds like that must have been terrible," I say, shaking my head. My words do not convey the emotion I feel. I look at her. Her blue shirt is hanging from her shoulders as she sits slumped over. "How are you feeling now?" I ask.

"Better. It don't hurt no more." Her voice has slowed, she is speaking softly now, looking down at the ground. Then she looks toward the door. "I don't know what to do. I don't know when he is going to hit me again. He's acting fine now. Bought me a new red coat. Maybe he realizes what a stupid thing that was, getting upset over dinner like that." She pauses, looks off to the side thoughtfully, then continues, "I should not have let dinner be so late that night, but I had to do the shopping after work, and there was a long line at the checkout counter. From now on I'll leave more time." She hesitates, looks straight at me, and continues, "I don't want you getting the wrong impression. He's a good man, it's just . . . sometimes he gets . . . well . . . angry. I don't know why. Maybe it's his upbringing. His dad was an alcoholic. I'm afraid, though; I don't know when it's going to happen again. If I watch myself, and keep things around the house real good . . . maybe he realized now; he is acting nice. . . . Maybe he ain't going to do nothing like that again."

I try to think how I can explain abuse so that Lucretia will understand. I learned about spouse abuse, or domestic violence, as a part of my residency in family medicine. I want her to see that what she is living through is not at all her fault, and that things will not get better by her hoping they will, or by her doing her errands more carefully. She will either need to sever this relationship or somehow convince both herself and her boyfriend to get extensive psychological help; otherwise, she will find herself living through a pattern of abuse that will repeat itself in a series of roller-coaster ups and downs, where the downs will become more dangerous while the ups will remain deceptively smooth and safe.

We talk for about twenty minutes. She is thinking of leaving her boyfriend but she has no place to go. She feels trapped. She cares for him and isn't sure that she wants to leave him. Perhaps, she says, they can work things out. I try to point out to her that, if she wants, there is a way out. Yet I realize that she cannot just walk away; rather, her situation is like that of a wolf caught in a trap—before the wolf walks, or limps, away, it must chew off its leg and leave a large part of itself permanently behind. To decide to go through such pain in order to live takes an enormous instinct for survival. I can only hope to tap some instinct that may still lie deep inside her, whispering with a small voice for her to save herself and her child. I can only plant an idea, tell her that options are available, so that as she thinks about her situation, she will be aware that there is help available if she chooses to seek it.

I give her the phone number of a local organization for women who are in abusive relationships. The organization provides professional counseling and can set up temporary living arrangements. I warn her not to think that things have suddenly changed because he bought her a red coat and is treating her well this week. I explain that after a man beats a woman, he often feels guilty and may try to treat her especially well for a while. Usually, though, the beatings start again. "Has he abused your son at all?" I ask. Half of the men who batter their wives also beat their children.

"No. He's yelled at him some, but he ain't never hit him. My son used to like him, but no more. Now he just tries to stay away from him." She moves nervously in her chair, rubbing her hands on her legs. She continues, "I also been talking to his mother. She says he's on the verge of a nervous breakdown, and if I leave him then she is sure that will be the end of him. That he may go crazy. I can't do that to him."

"Would his nervous breakdown be your fault?" I ask. She is taking responsibility for his problems. She is feeling guilty for his inability to cope, for his mental illness, and by extension, is feeling partly responsible for the way he abuses her. As long as she takes responsibility for his actions as well as her own, he will not have to take responsibility for his actions, and it is unlikely that their situation will improve.

She shifts again in her chair. "I don't know. I don't know whose fault it is. Some of it's mine. Some of it's his, I guess." Her eyes are red and watery and she wipes her right eye with her shirt sleeve. Then she looks nervously toward the door. "He's waiting for me outside and he'll be wondering what took so long. Please take the stitches out. I need to go."

I pick up the scissors and forceps. "I'd like you to come back in a week so we can talk some more," I say, knowing it's unlikely she will return. I tilt her head back and focus the examination light over the wound. Her scalp is shining in the light. Silently, one at a time, I grasp each suture, slide my scissors in, snip, and pull the suture out. I deposit each one in the plastic tray. It takes me about five minutes. Then I push the examination lamp away and step back.

"Your scar looks good," I tell her. "Once your hair grows around it no one will even know it's there."

She mumbles thanks, grabs her coat, and walks out of the room.

I stare at the doorway she just passed through. From the hallway I hear, "What took so long, Cretia?" "Don't know," she replies. "Doctor said one of them things was stuck in there real far."

It Floats in a Pain
That Needs a Body

THE WAITING ROOM was filled with patients as I walked through the front door. I was forty-five minutes late starting afternoon office hours, my shoes and socks were wet, and my pants were soaked to the knee after walking ten blocks from the hospital to our office in the March rain. Morning hospital rounds had been busy, and I wanted to take a minute to go back to the consultation room, hang up my coat, and take a deep breath. It was one fifteen and I needed to be back at the hospital by four o'clock.

"Doctor, it's for you," Janet, the nurse, called to me, looking up from the phone as I walked past her down the hall. Then she put her hand over the mouthpiece of the phone, "Do you know a Megan Gulligen?"

I shook my head. I threw my wet coat over a chair and leaned my umbrella against the nurses' station.

"Well, you're her doctor, and it's the twelfth time that she's called in the past hour." Janet rolled her eyes. "I asked her to make an appointment but she doesn't want to. She wants to talk to the doctor, right now."

"Get her number and I'll call her back in five minutes," I said.

"She doesn't have a number, she says. She's at a pay

phone." Janet seemed to be enjoying how disheveled I looked as she handed me the phone.

Before I could say hello the woman on the phone began, "Ohhh, Doctor . . . ohh Doctor . . . I'm in so much pain. Do something. Have compassion toward an old woman. I'm frail. I'm not strong like I used to be. Help me, Doctor . . ." I looked up at Janet, who was standing, smiling, and leaning against the desk.

"What seems to be the prob . . ." Ms. Gulligen started talking again before I could finish my sentence.

"Three days now I've been hurting. No one wants to help me, no one cares. Ohhh . . ." her voice bleated like a goat caught in a picket fence, "Ohhh, no one cares. The pain I kept hidden for so long. No one wants to help me. Do something. Do something for me, please!"

I put my hand over the receiver and asked for Ms. Gulligen's chart. Janet told me that we did not have an office chart for Ms. Gulligen. She had signed up to recieve her medical care from our office through the city's medical assistance program. On paper, we were her primary care physicians, responsible for all of her medical care, but we had never met her.

"What seems to be the *main* problem?" I asked.

"The pain! I told you that! Do I need more problems? Do I need more people asking me questions? I have pain flowing through my body. It's a terrible pain! Don't you believe me? Do something for me!"

"Where are you hurting most?" I asked her, watching Janet weigh Mrs. Chester, a three-hundred-thirty-pound middle-aged woman with diabetes who comes to the office once a month for nutritional counseling and to have her blood pressure checked.

"What do you mean, where do I hurt!" Ms. Gulligen responded. "All doctors ask the same stupid questions. I'm in pain! You're the doctor. You know where my pain is. I have pain all over. Every part of my body eats into me like frogs. God, please, help me." She was sobbing. I heard a police siren in the background, and what sounded like a train. She was probably calling from a pay phone under the el in the north part of the city.

"It's hard for me to hear you with all the noise in the background. Where are you?" I asked.

"I'm in the northeast, across from the emergency center," she sobbed, her deep breaths making it difficult for me to understand her. "They saw me in emergency yesterday. They won't see me again. . . . They said there's . . . there's nothing wrong with me . . . but I know there is. . . . I know there is something wrong . . . with me. There is something terribly . . . terribly wrong with me. If there was nothing wrong with me . . . I wouldn't be in pain. . . . Tell me, Doctor . . . why would I be in such pain?"

I felt like hanging up. Between the train in the background and her inability to state any more specifically what was bothering her, I did not think spending more time on the phone would be productive. And I was getting further behind with the patients who were already waiting here in the office. "Why don't you come into the office and let me examine you?" I asked.

"I can't get there," she said, and started sobbing again. "I don't have money for a cab. I cannot walk, my feet hurt me too much. I have bunions, and it's raining out. Please come see me. . . . I'll wait here for you. . . . I can pay you. . . . I'll wait across the street in the donut shop. It's a nice donut shop. You'll like it. I'll buy you a donut, you can give me medicine for my pain."

"I can't go to see you and I don't know how you can get here," I snapped. "If you get here in the next hour, I'll be happy to see you. Otherwise . . ."

"My pain," she cut me off again. "I don't know how I can get there." She cried out, "Ohhh . . ." Then the line went dead.

Two hours and eight patients later I was in the middle of examining a young woman with asthma, when Janet burst into the exam room. "Doctor, come quick," she said. "A patient just walked off the elevator and fainted."

I followed her down the hall to the waiting room. Slumped back on a chair in the middle of the waiting room was a middle-aged woman with eyes shut and a bright red wig hanging off her head. The wig was pinned between her head, which was flung back, and the wall supporting her head. Her thin gray hair was visible around the right edge of the wig. She was wearing a green paisley dress and had three large green emerald rings on her right hand, which was lying across the chair next to her. On the ring finger of her left hand was a big red ruby in an elaborate setting. Her left hand was lying across the back of the chair on her left side. Her fingernails were painted light blue and her makeup was caked on as if she were in a Broadway musical, which, I suspected, she might sometimes have thought she was in.

I walked over to her, observing that she was breathing,

and that the rise and fall of her chest was soft and regular. Fainting is usually due to a person's blood pressure dropping to a point where the pressure generated by the body is not great enough to move blood against gravity from the heart to the brain. This woman did not look like a person who has fainted—those people are usually pale and sweaty, and are certainly not posed with arms widespread.

"Wake up," I said, loudly, placing my hand on her left shoulder. I began shaking her. Her head jiggled and her wig dropped to the floor.

She didn't move.

I placed one hand on each padded shoulder of her dress. "Wake up," I repeated, shaking her back and forth more vigorously.

She still didn't move. I wondered if my assessment that this was not a true blackout was wrong. At the same time, I preferred not to become a part of her charade if she was faking.

I asked Janet to hand me the blood pressure cuff, rolled up the woman's polyester dress sleeve, and wrapped the rubber cuff around the loose, dry skin of her upper arm.

Her blood pressure was 130/76, normal, which strongly suggested that her lack of responsiveness was not from lack of perfusion of her brain with blood. Her pulse and respiration were normal rate and rhythm. A quick listen to her heart and lungs sounded fine.

I asked the people in the waiting room if she had had a seizure. She had not. I wondered if she might be diabetic, in a coma from low blood sugar, but she did not look pale or sweaty.

I played my hunch.

"We don't see people in this office who are blacked out," I said loudly into her ear. "People who black out we send to the emergency room. If you want to be seen here you are going to have to wake up, now. If not, we will get an ambulance to take you away."

I stepped back and watched her.

First her neck began to twitch, then her shoulders. She started moving her eyebrows up and down. Then opened one eye.

"Huh . . . what's that? Your wha . . . you whaa . . . what!?" She started mumbling and began rolling both eyes toward the ceiling.

"I said wake up or we're sending you to the ER. Those are the rules here."

She mumbled incoherently, then sat bolt upright and stared straight at me. Her eyes turned into narrow slits and her right hand began shaking.

"I came all this distance to be seen," she said. "I have pain deep inside of me. You are my doctor."

"I know," I said. "Are you Ms. Gulligen?"

She tilted her head, smiled, and batted her eyelashes. "Yes, I am. I am so glad I came here. I know you are a good doctor. You will cure my pain. I can tell from your eyes. They are like two bullets that shoot through my body to where the pain is. I promise you I won't black out anymore. It was the long walk, in the cold and the rain."

"It wasn't the cold or the rain. Why did you black out?" I asked, again playing my hunch, but being careful not to let my questions suggest to her what to say.

She smiled. "He told me to."

"Who?"

"The other doctor."

"What other doctor?"

"The doctor who did my hysterectomy three years ago." She paused. "He follows me."

"He follows you?"

"Yes."

"And he told you to black out?" I asked.

"Yes."

"Does he tell you to do other things?"

"He makes me take pills and then he wakes me up and torments me!" Her face became contorted and her voice rose to a shrill, high pitch. "He torments me and he twists my secret place. He twists it and sticks needles in it like I was a doll! Then he sprinkles powder outside my door and watches it seep into my room and make me itch." She put her head in her hands and started sobbing.

In the examination room Ms. Gulligen was wiping her eyes with a large green handkerchief. She had taken her shoes off and placed them in the sink. Her eyes had dark bags beneath them that were caked with makeup. As I walked in the room, she looked up, gave a meek smile, and started talking again, "You have to help me. I have so much pain. I know you think I'm a schizo, but I'm not. The doctor tried to give me pills and that's what caused this pain. I stopped taking the pills two months ago, but the pain is getting worse. You have to help me."

It sounded as if some physician had made the diagnosis of schizophrenia in the past and had given her antipsychotic medications to take to treat it. Then, as sometimes happens, she stopped taking her medicines, possibly because she began having paranoid delusions that the doctor was trying to hurt her and the medicines were causing her problems. Since she stopped taking her medications, her delusions and sense of paranoia had probably become worse.

One of the characteristics of untreated schizophrenia is delusions, which she was certainly displaying. She was imagining a doctor following her around, trying to give her pills and sticking pins in her. Also suggesting schizophrenia was her unusual affect and the bizarre imagery she used in describing the things that she felt were happening to her. At the same time, though, it was possible that not everything that she said was a product of her delusions, and it was very difficult to separate what was really happening to her from what she imagined to be happening to her.

It seemed very likely that Ms. Gulligen did have schizophrenia, and as a part of her mental illness had incorporated a physician she had seen three years ago, if such a person ever existed, as part of a paranoid delusional system that tormented her. In her original phone call she implied that she did not trust the assessment of the emergency physicians that she had seen the day before. It was unlikely that her visit with me would go much better.

Although I was confident that none of her previous doctors had tried to inflict pain on her, she was probably correct in feeling that they did not care very much about her. Schizophrenic patients, because of their unusual manner, their difficulty in carrying on normal conversations, and their unusual body postures, do not evoke a strong caring response in most people—physicians included. The old saying, Just because you're paranoid doesn't mean that people aren't out to get you, is sometimes not far from the truth.

"Where is your pain?" I asked.

"Why does everyone ask the same questions? Why doesn't anyone want to help me? I have pain all over, can't you see? Help me." Then she continued in a controlled voice. "I worked in a hospital once. I worked for one of the best surgeons in the city. He told me that I was one of the brightest girls working for him. He told me that I had a future in medicine. Don't ask me silly questions about pain, Doctor. I took care of patients so I know what I'm talking about." She pointed her finger at me. "Tell me what's wrong with me. I'm hurting."

Persons with schizophrenia may also believe that other people can read their thoughts. If she believed that, then it made sense that my questions would upset her. Since I already knew her feelings, my questions were further proof that I didn't care about her and that I was choosing to taunt instead of treat her. "Why don't you have a seat on the examination table?" I asked her.

She stuffed the handkerchief back in her pocket, fixed her dress, and walked to the table.

"Now show me where it hurts," I asked again. She was calmer now.

"Everywhere. My feet, my stomach, my back, my head. Oh, I have got a headache." She started rummaging through her large pocketbook. Smiling and cocking her head back she continued, "Dr. Gilfinkle . . . oh . . . I shouldn't tell you his name . . . I promised I wouldn't tell . . . has been sneaking pills into my handbag. The pills make smoke that seeps through my handbag. I see the vapors at night. The vapors look so soft, but they float in a pain that needs a body. When they touch my body they start a fire burning in me!"

I asked her to put on an examination gown and attempted to do a physical exam. I placed the ophthalmoscope near her eyes and she jerked her head away, saying the light hurt her. I tried to examine her eardrums, and she pushed my hand away as the scope touched her ear canal. I placed my stethoscope against her chest to listen to her breath sounds. After two full, clear, breaths, she shrieked out in pain, amplified a hundredfold through my stethoscope. I placed my hand on her shoulder and she yelped in pain. I brushed her elbow with my hand and she pushed my hand away. It hurt when I touched her fingers or toes. There was absolutely no way I could get any useful information from her physical exam. It appeared that she needed psychiatric care and needed to be on medications for schizophrenia.

I stepped back.

"What is it?" she asked, looking at me with empty eyes. "What do I have? Give me a pill for this pain. It's so awful." She held her emerald-studded right hand to her head in a dramatic gesture.

"It's not clear to me what's causing your pain," I tried to explain. "But clearly you're hurting. What I'd like to do is get a psychiatric opinion to see if there is a medicine that can help you to focus better so you can describe to me what is hurting. That would help me figure out where your pain is coming from, and then hopefully I will be able to help you."

"They will give me red pills. They gave me them the last time they saw me." Her voice rose and a look of terror came into her eyes. "I'm not taking the red pills again! That's what started my problems twenty years ago. I was a nurse's aide until I started the red pills." She trembled and bit her lip. Then she tilted her head up in a gesture of pride, and her wig slid partway off on her head, exposing her gray hair. "I'm not going to a psychiatrist; they're all crazier than I am."

"They're not *all* crazier," I replied, smiling. "You need psychiatric treatment. I can't help your pain until you get that treatment. I'd be happy to call the psychiatric center to arrange for you to be seen."

"I will not . . ."

"That's all we can do for . . ."

"I will not go to see any psychiatrist. I refuse to . . ."

"That's your decision," I said. "My recommendation is that you see a psychiatrist. Think about it. I'll be back in five minutes."

I left the room without waiting for a response. I was upset that I was now going to be late for afternoon rounds at the hospital, but satisfied with the way I had handled things—that I had not let myself be drawn into a half-hour discussion that would have gone nowhere.

Looking out the window in the consultation room, watching the cool March rain continue to fall, my mind wandered back to nine months ago when I had started in this office. How would I have handled Ms. Gulligen then? Would I have spent more time with her? Would I have tried harder to figure out what was wrong? I probably would have let her ramble on more, though I don't think I would have been better at ferreting out her problems, and I would have ended up further behind than I was now. Though spending more time in the room with her would not have helped, the fact that I was now able to cut her off in the middle of her sentence and walk out of the room bothered me.

I glanced at my watch. It was three forty-five. I was due

back at the hospital at four o'clock. I began to see the patients who were left in the office. The woman with asthma responded to medication and, after writing a prescription for her, I sent her home with instructions to follow up in the office in one week. The last two patients of the day had sore throats for which I prescribed antibiotics. Ms. Gulligen remained in her examination room, sitting with her arms folded over her chest. Janet worked on cleaning up the nurses' station and on some paperwork that she needed to complete from the past week. I walked back to the consultation room and stared out the window at the droplets of rain on the glass pane and the glaze the wetness left on the brick of the building. I wondered how many doctor's offices Ms. Gulligen had been to in the last few months, seeking relief from pains that never left her, refusing psychiatric treatment. Eventually she would probably walk into some poor physician's office having a heart attack, and it would be necessary, but next to impossible, for the physician to sense that her chest pain was the one thing he or she needed to focus on within the thicket of her other complaints. I wondered if today was that day, and if I was not fulfilling my responsibility to her because I was unable to break through the morass of her funny mind to figure out what was wrong.

I walked back to Ms. Gulligen's room. I stood and looked at her from the doorway. Her red wig was hanging halfway over her head, and she was playing with a tassel on her handbag.

"Well?" I said.

"I'm not moving until you give me medicine for this pain," she replied, her voice tired.

"First I need to know what is causing the pain, and I don't really think I'm going to be able to figure that out until you receive psychiatric care."

She sat on her chair looking at me nervously, then she began rolling her tongue over her upper lip and her right cheek started twitching. Her eyes grew wide and she raised her voice. "I'm not going to see some crazy psychiatrist," she said, and then, like a foghorn calling for a lost ship on a foggy night, "I'm in paaaaaaaain!"

I was unsure what to do. I needed to go back to the hospital. I did not want to spend an hour trying to convince her to receive psychiatric treatment, particularly since I didn't think she would ever agree with me.

"You have a choice. You can go the psychiatrist, and I'll be happy to get him to see you right away; we can arrange for a cab voucher that will pay for the cab to take you to the psychiatric center. Or you can get up and walk out of this office. The office is closing."

"I'm not leaving," she said, shaking her head. "You're the doctor and you're not taking care of me. You are supposed to make me better." She pulled a red handkerchief out of her pocketbook and blew her nose.

I walked back down the hall to the consultation room, put on my coat, and gathered my papers, hoping that by example I could encourage her to leave. Then I walked back to Ms. Gulligen's room.

"Ready to go?" I said.

"I'm not leaving," she growled, folding her arms tighter across her chest. "I watch TV and radio and I know my rights. Phil Donahue told me last week on TV that patients have rights, that they should make demands from their doctors. You can be sued if you don't help me. I know that. I used to work for the city." She stared at me. Her eyes were wide and bloodshot. Then she started banging her fist against the examination table, yelping, "I'm in pain, I'm in pain, I'm in pain. . . ."

I couldn't listen any more. I walked out of the room and down the hall again. Was I missing some important clue to her diagnosis? Did she really have a physical ailment? I had tried my best and she was impossible to talk to or examine. Or had I tried my best? Had I been distracted by how busy the day had been? Should I make one more attempt to take a medical history and examine her? It was unlikely that I would do any better than the first time I tried, and I was due back in the hospital twenty minutes ago. I had been in this office nine months and it was becoming increasingly clear to me that there were large barriers to the care I wanted to provide. These barriers presented themselves in different forms every day. I was unable to provide the quality of medical care I felt that my patients deserved, or at least the type of care I wanted to provide for them. I wondered if I could continue feeling this way over the next few months. I wondered if it was worth working here, if I was accomplishing anything, and how long I should continue despite the frustration.

I walked back to her room. She was sitting down again, with her arms folded and a washed-out look on her face. "I'm not leaving," she said flatly.

"Ms. Gulligen," I said, "if you don't leave now I'm going to have to call the police. The office closed an hour ago and it doesn't seem like we're getting anywhere."

She started banging the examination table with her hand

and screaming, "I will not leave. I know my rights. I'm in pain. I have such a pain. You are a mean, evil person. You're not a doctor, you're a devil. A devil is what you are. You are a devil, with hoofed feet. Help! Help! I'm being hurt by a devil and I'm in such pain! . . ."

I walked back to the hallway, picked up the phone, and called the police. Then I walked back to the consultation room to try to do some paperwork until the police came.

Ms. Gulligen and I stalked each other for the next half hour. I would sit in the consultation room attempting to look through lab tests as she was pacing up and down the hall, glancing in my room as she passed the door. If five minutes went by without her peeking in the door, I would get up, look in the examination room, and see her sitting, biting her fingernails, mumbling to herself, and shaking her head.

At the end of the half hour two policemen walked into the consultation room and asked me what the problem was. I explained and led them down the hall to Ms. Gulligen's examination room.

The door to the room was shut. I knocked twice and walked in. Lying on the crumpled paper of the examination table was a green handkerchief with gold embroidery. Her muddy black shoes were still in the sink.

Two weeks later I was poring over lab tests in the consultation room when Janet walked in and handed me a torn piece of paper with a note scribbled on it. We were being consulted, it said, for medical management of Megan Gulligen, admitted to the hospital earlier that morning for surgery on a perforated peptic ulcer.

The Street Sound Bar

THE PATIENTS KNOW the stories of the neighborhood. One patient, a man in his late sixties who has lived two blocks away from our office his whole life, told me about the night Billie Holiday, the great jazz and blues singer, sang in the bar that was now boarded up across the street from our office. That was in August 1956. He told me that some of the older people in the neighborhood still talk about it: the line of people reaching halfway around the block at two in the morning; the huge red neon sign, STREET SOUND BAR, that bathed the people and the block in phosphorescent light; the mugginess of the air; the cigarette smoke that was so dense you could barely see the jukebox from a seat near the bar; the yellowed light that filtered through the clouds of cigarette smoke; and the silence that came over the whole room when, at twenty minutes to three in the morning, Billie Holiday, the star whose life everyone in the room had read about and whose songs everyone had heard on the radio, walked softly onto the stage and began singing "Lady Sings the Blues."

That was back when this neighborhood offered some of the best jazz and blues to be found anywhere in the city. It offered the best of a number of other things as well, my patient said under his breath, with a chuckle. People used to stand in line for an hour to sit at a table and listen to music at the Street Sound Bar. Afterward they would walk down the block, have another drink, and listen to more jazz at one of the other clubs in the neighborhood.

The story of the neighborhood comes out in bits and pieces. It is told to me over time through chance conversations with patients. It is difficult for me to know what is truth and what is a product of memories. A middle-aged woman told me of how, in 1962, the city bureau of transportation announced their plan to run an extension of the interstate highway through the neighborhood, two blocks from the Street Sound Bar. She and some other members of the community banded together to try to stop construction of the highway. They collected a thousand signatures and sent them to the traffic commission. Hearings were set up in city hall. They even organized a small demonstration outside the mayor's office.

For two years their efforts delayed the construction of the highway. Finally, plans were changed and the highway was constructed three miles south of this neighborhood. Unfortunately, the damage had been done. While the tenants of the buildings were battling city hall, fighting for their homes and neighborhood, the landlords were trying to sell off their properties. The new owners did not care for the buildings the way the old owners had, and the old owners who couldn't find buyers became less and less willing to keep up buildings they were losing money on. This is one of the reasons why the neighborhood is in such bad shape, she told me.

A fifty-year-old man, a jazz saxophonist before his ear

went bad—from drinking too much alcohol and shooting too much dope, he says—told me about the Street Sound Bar in the 1960s. While the neighborhood was having its troubles, the Street Sound continued to play jazz and rock, but to smaller and smaller crowds. The tables that used to fill by eleven o'clock every night sat empty, and you could even get an open seat at the bar. The crowd that spent time in the bar changed in character. "A nice group of people," my patient said, "but they wasn't musicians the way the other folks was. So the musicians stopped coming. And the music lovers, they just went somewhere else."

Around 1965, "a year or so after the president was shot," the bar changed owners, though it kept the same name, and the thirty-foot-high red neon STREET SOUND BAR continued to shine from over the awning. For two years the new owner tried to revive the bar as a jazz club. He brought in the best talent in the city. It didn't work. My patient told me that the owner committed suicide in the back room of the top floor of the building, taking a handful of sleeping pills and washing them down with one of the bar's finest bottles of whiskey. The bar sat empty for a year, the unlit sign casting a long shadow on the dark street when the full moon shined. The club was sold at a bargain price, says my patient, and revived the next year, first as a jazz club, then a few months later as a cabaret/strip joint. It closed for the last time in 1969, the same year men walked on the moon.

Last week was the first week of spring. I have been in this office a little over nine months and I feel as if an understanding, of my patients and their lives, has slowly grown inside of me. I am not sure how long I will remain here, how long I will choose to tolerate the frustration and sadness I feel over the limits to the care I can provide. Lately, though, I have also felt a sense of closeness to my patients; I have found myself able to communicate with them more easily. It is as if we have begun to understand each other, often before I even say hello. It is an understanding that goes beyond words, that precedes words.

Last week I looked out my office window and saw a man standing on the roof of the Street Sound Bar with a large sledge hammer. Toward the back of the building, also on the flat tar roof, were two other men. One was holding a crowbar. The other was leaning on the long wooden handle of an axe, the metal part of the axe resting on the roof. Down below, two men were dragging a yellow barricade into the middle of the street to divert traffic. The man at the front of the roof, standing right at the roof's edge, looked down toward the enormous, rusted, thirty-foot sign that said STREET SOUND BAR, in chipped paint and brown glass. The sign was attached by rusted metal posts bolted into the red brick of the building at the level of the first story and just above the fourth story, below the roof.

The man held the sledge hammer over the side of the roof, letting it sway in his hands like a pendulum marking time. His muscles stood out from the thin, sleeveless gray T-shirt he was wearing as the morning sun shined on him. He looked down one more time, then raised the large metal hammer high above his head. As the hammer was suspended in the air, the two men toward the back of the roof seemed motionless; no cars or people moved in the street below. Then the hammer made a smooth arc through the air till it landed, with a crash, on the upper metal post, bounced back, and hit the post a second time. The man raised his hammer again and let it crash down against the post. A crack developed in the brick wall. He lifted his hammer again, and let it crash into the post, and again, sweat flying from him, and again, and again. The post moved away from the brick wall, and the sign began to sag. He lifted the hammer again, and let it crash. The metal post separated from the brick. The enormous sign, held to the wall only by its lower post, then buckled under its own weight, and began to fall from the wall. For a moment its descent was halted by the lower post, which seemed to refuse to give up the heritage it had supported for twenty-five years. Then, bending under the weight of time and gravity, the post snapped, and the sign crashed to the ground.

I have watched these men, every morning and afternoon for the last week, from the window of my office, as they slam hammers and axes into the wood and brick of the building, crumpling walls, floors, and ceilings.

During the last week the crew demolished the top floor of the building, and now the third floor lies exposed. From my window, I can see into each separate room. I watch the men swing sledge hammers at the walls and toss pieces of wood over the side onto a growing pile three stories below. One man, in a room toward the front, tries to pry loose a wooden beam that is lying on the floor. It doesn't come easily away from the clutter that surrounds it. He pulls it and pulls it and it comes loose, a piece of dirty linen hanging from its end like a tattered flag. The piece of linen suggests what might have gone on in the privacy of the rooms upstairs from the bar. Lifting the heavy beam, the man readjusts his weight, holding the beam at an angle from the floor, its yellow sheet dangling. The scene looks like the famous sculpture at Iwo Jima, where five men, in the mist of battle, raise a flag out of the dirt. Arching his back, he hoists the beam up and over the side of the building to go crashing three stories into a pile of trash on the sidewalk below.

The top two stories of the building are now demolished and I can see clear across to the next street. Behind the building smoke rises, like the smoke that used to rise years ago from cigarettes held in the hands of hundreds of people dressed for an evening of jazz and blues, and whatever action came their way. The smoke now rises from a pit where men in hardhats toss wood from the building they are ripping apart. One man is smoking a cigarette while tending the fire in the pit. I wonder if he grew up nearby. Could he be thinking of the grandness of the building that is disintegrating in the flames? Could both of us, separately, be sharing similar thoughts of how much our society has changed in the last thirty years, of how much we all have advanced, and how it becomes more clear, with each panel that is torn from this building and thrown into the fire, how much we have lost and are losing?

There is an abandoned building next door to the Street Sound Bar. The front entrance to the building is bolted by a long iron bar that crosses the width of the door frame. There is a thick padlock on each end of the rusted bolt. The windows of the building have been covered with thick wooden boards and sheets of aluminum. In the evenings this past winter, when I walked out of my office, I could see thin rays of light creeping through slits at the edges of the boarded-up windows in the basement. I wondered if the light was from a homeless person who had set up shelter there, finding his or her way in through a hole in the back of the building, lighting the abandoned room with a kerosene lamp or an old flashlight, or simply with a fire in a tin drum. Or, I wondered, was the light coming from enterprising members of the community, selling cocaine, amphetamines, or heroin from a protected bower across from our medical office? I wonder if that person is still there this spring, if he or she sleeps in the basement during the day, and how the hammering and crashing of debris must be disturbing.

The man with the hardhat, standing by the fire, takes one last deep drag on his cigarette and tosses it into the flames. He bends over the woodpile and pulls out a long piece that is about as wide as a man's hand and six feet long with a series of diamonds carved into it. The wood is covered with chipped maroon paint, and I recognize it as the border of the roof, another detail indicating the attention the builders must have paid to the appearance of the building, another detail that helped the Street Sound Bar stand out among the other buildings in this once-thriving neighborhood. The man with the yellow hardhat jerks the piece of wood from the pile and, swinging it from his hip, heaves it into the fire.

The construction workers are now gone. The building lies in a heap of brick, wire, and burned wood. I see a black cat cross carefully over the rubbish, balancing on a long rotted beam that lies suspended between a pile of bricks and the broken doorway to which it used to be connected. An old man, wearing a black suit with sleeves that are too long for him and a gray cap, walks bent over with the aid of a cane. He walks slowly and carefully on the sidewalk in front of the wreckage, avoiding any wood or brick in his path. A young boy, about five years old, wearing a red baseball cap and a blue zippered jacket with an orange New York Mets logo sewn on its back, is playing in the front corner of the lot. He picks up a shattered piece of glass, perhaps the only remnant of the grand mirror that was behind the bar. As he turns the piece of glass over in his hand, it reflects a broken glint of the brilliant spring sun.

The Sultan

WE WERE BUSIER than usual for August, partly I believe, because our waiting room was air conditioned and most of the neighborhood was not. For nearly two months the sun had been beating down on the parched streets during the day, and its heat had been radiating up from the dark pavements at night. There had been no rain, the city's water supplies were dangerously low, and there was no relief in sight.

I stood at the end of the hall and looked out the window of our third-story office at the projects down the block. I had been at this office over a year and the sights from this window were becoming familiar. In the courtyard and the street by the projects crowds of people were walking languorously about, leaning on cars, fanning themselves, and talking. At the far end of the courtyard children were running in and out of the spray from an opened fire hydrant. Four old women sat watching, on folding aluminum chairs in the shade of the tall building, fanning themselves with paper plates and newspapers. I turned from the window to see Mr. Stewart, wearing a wide-brimmed straw hat with a thick yellow band around it, being led by the nurse down the hall to the examination room.

I wiped some sweat from my forehead, walked down

the hall, and picked up his chart. He was a new patient to the office, come in because of dizziness, which seemed to be the complaint of the summer. When I walked into the examination room he took off his hat and extended his hand.

"How are ya, Doc?" he said, a hint of a smile on his face. His voice was smooth and calm; beads of sweat glistened on his chest and forehead. He had a lanky build, was in his mid-sixties, with balding gray hair and a patchy beard, and he was wearing a red-and-white checkered shirt open to mid-chest. His shoes were a size or two too big for him, leaving a noticeable gap behind his heels, but they were well polished and pointed at the toe. His smile broadened, exposing big yellow teeth. It was a smile that said that he was comfortable with himself and others, a friendly smile, the kind that comes from a long distance to slide up real close. As his eyes roamed over me like a boxer assessing his opponent—not, I believe, necessarily because he didn't trust me, but because it was his habit to get to know people quickly—he continued, "Heat enough for you today?"

I nodded and introduced myself as we shook hands. Then he leaned back in the chair, and I sensed that I had passed his test, whatever it was.

"Been reeeaaal hot out lately, don't ya think?" he said, then he paused and looked up at the ceiling. "I been having some trouble walking. My feet just seem to go out on me. Real unsteady-like."

"Have a seat on the examination table," I told him.

He lifted his spindly body from the chair, holding the examination table with one hand to steady himself. Then he got up on the exam table and stared straight ahead as if he were facing a firing squad.

I mechanically went through Mr. Stewart's exam. I expected the same exam I had been seeing two or three times a day that summer on people who had been coming in lightheaded: normal blood pressure taken with them lying and standing, normal retina exam, and a normal neurologic exam. All leaving me with the same conclusion: mild dehydration due to the oppressive heat. On Mr. Stewart's exam, though, I was unable to elicit any reflexes in his knees or ankles. I asked him to take off his shoes and socks so I could examine him further. I took one of his large toes between the thumb and forefinger of my right hand. The skin was thin and a flaking yellow nail curved over the front of the toe.

"I am going to move your toe," I told him. "Without looking, tell me whether I move it up or down." I moved his toe slightly toward the ceiling.

His face wrinkled with concentration.

I moved the toe up a little more.

"Can you tell me which way I moved your toe?" I asked.

He looked puzzled and disturbed.

"I . . . I'm not sure, Doc. Down? . . . Or up? I don't know."

"Now?" I moved the toe up far toward the ceiling.

"No," he replied, shaking his head.

I let go of his toe and moved his ankle. He could sense gross movement, but could not tell when I only moved his ankle slightly. I sat up in my chair.

"Do you drink alcohol, Mr. Stewart?" I asked him.

"I drink my share," he said with assurance, and smiled.

"What kind?" I asked.

"Moonshine. Good moonshine. My friend's cousin brings

it up, about once a month, from North Carolina." He leaned back, looked up at the ceiling for a moment, then back at me with a big smile. "You ever taste moonshine? They don't make stuff like that in the north."

"About how much moonshine do you drink?" I couldn't help smiling back at him.

"Oh, not that much." He crossed his legs and cupped his hands on each other over his thigh. His eyes twinkled. "A few shots. Maybe a fifth now and then when me and the boys get together."

I looked at him and began to think of the diseases that might explain his problem. He had lost the ability to tell where his feet were. That meant that something had destroyed the capacity of his peripheral nerves to transmit information about leg position back to his brain. It could have been long years of drinking moonshine that caused this, the alcohol acting like an anesthetic, bathing his nerve endings through the years until they were dulled permanently to the sensations of his own body. Or it could have been due to lead, a neurotoxin that often leaches into moonshine from the lead solder connecting the pipes that the alcohol vapor passes through on its way from cornmeal to brew. Many other possible causes existed as well.

"Did you ever get a shot for any disease?" I asked.

"A long time ago. When I was in prison, back in the sixties. I got a wicked shot in my butt. An ugly doctor with pockmarks gave me the shot. His face made my butt look good." He leaned his head back and laughed, rocking his whole body. "He said I had the clap."

"OK," I said, thinking. "Let's draw some blood tests and I'd like to see you back in the office in a week. In the meantime, I want you drinking lots of water. Don't let this weather get to you, OK?"

Mr. Stewart missed his appointment. Perhaps his unsteadiness improved with the break in the weather, perhaps he just forgot, or had something else to do. His blood tests came back to the office indicating that he had been infected with syphilis. I couldn't tell from the test result whether he had syphilis that had already been treated, or whether he was recently infected. It was possible that the treatment he had received thirty years ago did not adequately treat the infection, which had lain dormant for thirty years and now was beginning to cause his symptoms. In order to determine what was going on, Mr. Stewart would need further tests, most importantly, a spinal tap. Only by taking cerebrospinal fluid out of his spinal canal and testing it for syphilis could we tell if his present symptoms were due to syphilis.

I got out his medical chart and dialed his number. The phone was disconnected, so I sent a letter to him explaining that he had a serious infection that would require treatment and that he should contact our office immediately.

Ten days later the letter returned to us stamped in red ink that no such address existed. The postman told us that the address we sent the letter to was a demolished building. I returned the letter to his chart, sent a photocopy of the letter with a note attached about our inability to contact him to the city's department of health, and returned the chart to the file cabinet.

Looking out the window of my office at the brick building across the street and the children playing jump rope on the sidewalk, I thought that in some corner of the city, Mr.

Stewart was probably playing cards, slapping a woman on the thigh, and drinking moonshine whiskey with his buddies while microscopic spiral-shaped organisms were swirling round and round in the eddy of his cerebrospinal fluid, making a meal of his brain.

It was snowing. I was telling the receptionist that we were going to close the office early because of the ice when an older man limped off the elevator. He was wearing a long blue wool overcoat covered with snow and a wide-brimmed leather hat. He looked around the room, brushed the snow off his coat, shook his head, then walked over to me in the waiting room.

"Doc," he said, removing his overcoat to reveal a smaller red coat underneath. "That dizziness is still there. It's getting worse, you know, you gotta do something for me." He took his hat off and held it in the same hand as his coat. He had three weeks' growth of stubbly beard and worried bloodshot eyes set in deep bags of skin.

"Where have you been the last six months?" I asked. "I tried sending you a letter, but you gave us a fake address."

"Oh, that's no fake address." He chuckled. "There's just no building there anymore. I always use that address."

He paused for a moment, then continued. "I been busy, taking care of some things. Then I was feeling OK for a while, you know, better. I tried taking herbs. But then it start coming back again. Don't know where it come back from. Even the herbs don't work no more."

"Why don't we have the nurse put you back in an examination room and I'll take a look at you," I said. So much for closing the office early. I went to the window and watched the snow falling. There was about four inches of snow on the ground. It made the streets look clean, almost pure, and muffled the incessant drone of the traffic one block away on Broad Street.

In the examination room, Mr. Stewart was sitting on the table wearing an examination gown. His skin looked leathery and wrinkled. "Tell me what's been going on," I asked.

"Well, I been busy, I been real busy. I been trying to ignore it, but this thing, it keeps getting worse, you know. Don't know what it is. I getting dizzy all the time now. And I ain't remembering things. I mean bad. Real bad. Like I was eating chicken the other night. And I ate this whole drumstick and a wing. It was a big piece." He held his hands about six inches apart, showing me the size of the piece of chicken. "Then, fifteen minutes later, I'm sitting with my friend Ralph, and I asked Ralph why we wasn't being given anything to eat. He looked at me like I was crazy; he said what's I talking out of my head for, we just finished eating. I said what you lying to me for, you my best friend, and he goes to the trash can and pulls out the chicken bones."

"That sounds bad. Have you noticed anything else?" I asked.

"Well, I'm losing control of my pee sometimes." He looked up at me. "What's going on?"

"Remember you told me you were treated for clap?"

"Yeah."

"Well, it could still be in your system, causing all your problems. The only way to know is to check your spinal fluid for syphilis." I looked straight at him staring straight at me. He did not trust people easily, and I could tell he was considering whether or not he should trust me.

"How do you do that?" he asked, squinting and leaning forward.

"We would need to do a spinal tap. That means putting a needle through your back into the fluid around your spinal cord," I told him.

He raised his eyebrows. "It hurt?"

"A little, not much. We can numb up the area first. I want you to get a CAT scan of your head before we do the tap." I had to make sure that his symptoms were not being caused by an unusual brain tumor. If we did a spinal tap with a tumor present, the otherwise simple procedure could be complicated by increased pressure from the tumor causing the contents of the brain to be pushed into the spinal canal.

He agreed to do whatever we recommended to help him find out why he was dizzy and losing his memory. I asked the nurse to schedule the CAT scan and gave him an appointment to see us for the spinal tap once the scan was done.

It was early spring and the sun was shining. The tree that grew from a square of soil in the sidewalk in front of our office was beginning to bloom. The pigeons were squawking more than usual, and people were out milling about the street and courtyard, when Mr. Stewart, wearing an oversized coat and well-polished shoes, teetered in looking even more washed out than the last time I had seen him.

"Doc, you gotta help me," his eyes were wide and worried as he turned back to look at me while the nurse led him down the hall to the examination room.

I lifted his chart from the desk and walked dully across the hall and into the examination room. Mr. Stewart looked as if he had been through war. "What's been going on?" I asked him.

"My dizziness is getting worse all the time, and I ain't barely got no memory left," he told me.

"If it's been that bad, why did you miss the appointment for the CAT scan and then not show up here for four months?"

"I don't know, something came up, or something. I need some help, Doc, I'm serious. I don't know how I can keep on living like this." He was shaking his head. The smell of alcohol floated across the room.

"How much have you been drinking?" I asked.

"Oh . . ." he paused, looked up at the ceiling, then back at me. "I ain't been drinking all that much. About a fifth a whiskey a day. But only when I have the money."

"What other drugs are you doing?"

"None, really. . . . Ain't skin-popped in a week," he replied. He shook his head, belched, then shook his head some more. At least he was being honest with me. Maybe.

I thought for a minute about how to get the tests that he needed done and whether to try ordering the CAT scan again, hoping he would show up for it this time since he seemed more worried. I decided that his potential diagnosis, syphilis that was eating away at his brain, was a serious enough problem that I needed to be sure that the tests got done.

"We should admit you to the hospital and get the tests we need nice and quick and easy. How's that sound to you?" I asked.

He stared at me with frightened eyes.

"Whatever you say, Doc. I'll do whatever you say," he responded, then bent over and placed his head in his hands.

Mr. Stewart enjoyed being in the hospital. Late on the afternoon of his admission the nurses nicknamed him the Sultan for the way he tied three hospital gowns around his torso making a robe and one around his head, the end flowing over his neck and back, resembling a turban. He spent most of the afternoon walking up and down the hall talking to staff and patients.

Mr. Stewart went for his CAT scan on the evening of his admission. It was normal. The next day the intern and I performed the spinal tap on him without problems and sent the clear cerebrospinal fluid to the lab for analysis. I thought about sending Mr. Stewart home and having him follow up the test results in the office, but decided not to. If the cerebrospinal fluid syphilis test was positive, I would have to admit him back to the hospital anyway. If I let him go home it might be a while until he came back for the results, if he came back at all.

"Isn't it a beautiful day out," Mr. Stewart said, perched on the windowsill at the end of the hallway, gazing out at the white magnolia trees in bloom every twenty feet along the sidewalk outside the hospital. "Haven't seen a day like this in years. Your people treat me real well here. I'll tell you, Doc, they treat me real well here." He smiled.

"I'm glad," I said, squinting in the sunlight coming through the picture window and reflecting off the waxed floors.

"How long you think I'll be able to stay here?" He tilted his head and raised his eyebrows. "Food's real good." Then he winked at me and nodded. He was looking fresher than he had in the office.

"Depends what your tests show. We should have them back by tomorrow. I'll talk to you then."

I walked down to the nurses' station. I opened his chart to write my daily note and found a letter from an administrator with the city health plan in the front of the chart. The chart had been reviewed, the letter said, and payment for all expenses related to Mr. Stewart's admission were being denied because there was insufficient reason for him to be in the hospital. The administrator's letter said that everything we were doing could have been done more easily and less expensively on an outpatient basis. I would have liked to see that administrator try to do tests on Mr. Stewart as an outpatient, ensure his follow-up, and be responsible for his care.

"Mr. Stewart's cerebrospinal fluid results just came back, and the result of the RPR [the rapid plasma reagin test for syphilis] was one to sixty-four," the nurse on the hospital floor for Mr. Stewart's room told me the next afternoon.

The test confirmed that Mr. Stewart had syphilis eating through his spinal cord and brain. In a way this was good news. He could be cured, or at least the progression of his disease could be halted, by treatment with ten days of intravenous penicillin.

I went downstairs to tell Mr. Stewart our findings. When I walked in his room I saw three hospital gowns lying on his bed. There was a half-filled pitcher of water and a crumpled pack of cigarettes on his dresser. The afternoon sun coming in through the window reflected off the cellophane wrapper of the cigarette pack. On the other side of the room I noticed one green hospital slipper leaning on its side against the wall. The other slipper was tucked halfway under the pillow at the head of the bed.

I walked out of the room and down the hall to Mr. Stewart's customary perch near the windowsill. Two hospital cleaning women were sitting on break talking. I went over to the next hall to see if he had found himself a new spot. He had not.

I found the nurse responsible for his care and asked her if she knew where he was. She had last seen him, she said, about an hour before, when he was mumbling something about how he was sick and tired of sitting around in a hospital while the doctors were making up their minds about what experiments to do on him next.

This was not the first time that I had heard one of my patients express concern about being experimented upon by a doctor. Among patients in the community I cared for, many viewed their doctors with suspicion, and though I tried to establish trust between myself and my patients, a lifetime of mistrust is not easily put aside. Unfortunately, this distrust is at least partially based on real events. Many medical studies have been done in inner-city hospitals that provide care for the poor, and patients or family members often have been asked to enroll in studies of new treatments or medications. Patients' views of the difference between being experimented upon and being enrolled in a study of a new medicine are often not the same as their physicians'. The most notorious instance of the medical establishment not fulfilling the trust society places in it occurred in Tuskegee, Alabama, where black men who were infected with syphilis were followed without being offered treatment in order to learn about the natural outcomes of untreated syphilis. This study, which ended in the early 1970s, was the impetus for many of the current ethical guidelines and safeguards that are in place to protect patients who are enrolled in research studies. Although this type of egregious research is no longer occurring, the mistrust that was generated as a result of early studies performed with poor ethical guidelines hovers over many physicians' attempts to establish bonds of trust with their inner-city patients.

The nurse and I walked to Mr. Stewart's room. I opened the drawer by his bed. It was empty. I opened his closet door. He had taken his clothes.

I looked at x-rays and checked labs for the next hour, taking care of some things that had to be done by the end of the afternoon and hoping that Mr. Stewart had gone out for a walk and might soon return. When he didn't, I went to his chart to see if he had given us a phone number to contact in case of an emergency. I dialed the number. It rang seven times and then a woman answered in a deep voice, "Oak and Hollow Lounge, can I help you?"

Oak and Hollow Lounge? I shook my head and thought for a moment, trying to place where I had heard the name before. I remembered. The Oak and Hollow Lounge was a run-down bar about five blocks from our office.

"This is a doctor from the hospital," I replied. "Do you know how I can get in touch with Edward Stewart?"

"No, I don't, I don't even know how to touch Edgewood Stert," she replied in a slurred voice that was nevertheless deep and appealing, then she laughed.

"Edward Stewart!" I repeated.

"Is he a friend of yours? I like men who look out for

their friends. A man who cares about his friends usually treats a woman real fine too." Her voice was sultry and exciting. I imagined her sitting languorously back in a tight black dress, one leg up on a wooden table, holding a cigarette in her left hand.

"He's not a friend," I said, snapping out of my daydream. "He's a patient and I'm his doctor. He gave us your number to contact for emergencies. Listen, he has a serious infection that may kill him if we don't get in touch. Why don't you help us? His name is Edward Stewart."

"That sounds real bad. Eddard Start? I . . . I don't . . . I don't know any Edge Start, but I'll tell *you* something baby, you got a real fine voice. I like your voice, so if you feel like having fun, why don't *you* come over and we'll see if you and I can have us a good time."

White Coat

"YOU GOTTA HELP me, Doc," Mr. Darron stammers as he stares past me like a shell-shocked soldier, his oily skin stretched thin over his face, a large purple vein pulsating on his forehead. He is sitting slumped over in a chair, leaning his left arm on the examination table. He has a week's growth of stubbly beard, his neck muscles are standing out, and his hair, usually perfectly styled and combed, is greasy and disheveled. "I don't know what's happening to me," he continues in a quavering voice. "I can't eat, I can't sleep, I feel nauseous all the time. The old lady's been nagging at me to get in to see ya. I feel goddamed awful."

Thursday afternoon office hours have begun, our busiest four hours each week. I readjust my white coat and button it in front of me as if it were armor. Mr. Darron does not have a scheduled appointment, but has come into the office today because he can no longer bear the way he feels. He goes on to tell me that for two months he has been feeling nauseated and extremely tired. In addition, he has begun to lose weight. Glancing at his medical chart, I see he has lost twenty pounds since his last office visit, four months ago. He doesn't explain anything more, just looks down while holding his head with his right hand. I have known

Mr. Darron for four years, taking care of him first during my internship and residency, and now as an attending physician. He is thirty-seven years old and has diabetes, high blood pressure, schizophrenia, and an intermittent problem with substance abuse. Over those four years I have taken care of him through three hospitalizations, two psychiatric admissions, and most of his regular outpatient visits. It hurts me to see him in this condition. I have seen how hard he works to try to keep his life together.

"Do you have pains anywhere?" I ask.

"No." He is now staring at the ground, pulling at his hair with his right hand.

"Any belly pain, chest pain, or difficulty swallowing?"

"Na. Nothing."

"Fevers?"

"No. I told you," he groans. "Just no energy, no zip. I don't feel like getting out of bed in the morning. And I feel so goddamed nauseous. I can't eat a thing."

I go on to take a complete history of his illness, including a discussion about alcohol and drug use. Then I perform a thorough physical exam. I am acutely aware that patients with scheduled appointments are getting annoyed outside at the lengthening wait. I keep to myself how upset I am that Mr. Darron has put off coming into the office for so long. I am upset both for him, because whatever is wrong with him has been continuing for longer than it needed to without medical attention, and for me, because his unscheduled visit is causing me to fall behind my afternoon schedule. I explain to Mr. Darron that I want to check a chest x-ray, samples of his stool for blood, and a number of blood tests, including a test for the AIDS virus, since he had used intravenous drugs in the past.

It takes me about an hour to perform a complete physical exam and explain my thoughts to Mr. Darron. He needs this hour of attention, but I wish he had called earlier in the week to make an appointment so that we could have put aside time for his exam. My scheduled patients have now been kept waiting an hour. When I walk out of the examination room I notice four charts in the bin, each one representing a patient waiting to be seen.

I walk down the end of the hall to the consultation room to take a deep breath and look out the window for a minute before going on to see the next patient. The room serves as a place of quiet retreat where I can go to gather my thoughts. I don't feel strong enough to see patients here today. The people I see have so much pain, and there is often so little that I feel I do for them. I have been at this office a year and a half now, and I question the value of what I am doing. Outside the window the few trees planted in the sidewalk sway in a strong December wind. In the vacant lot across the street a young boy has suspended a broken wooden beam between two cinder blocks. He is swaying with his arms extended as he balances, walking the length of the beam. A sheet of newspaper tumbles over and over the bricks and broken bottles and around the cinder blocks. In the far corner three old men sit and watch from metal folding chairs. On the block behind the vacant lot is an old stone Gothic church. Its majestic spire and dull stained glass seem to taunt what has become of this neighborhood.

I straighten out my white coat. In medical school we

were taught that doctors began to wear white coats in the early 1900s, with the general acceptance of the "germ theory of disease." The white coat, for patient and physician, indicated that the physician's dress was clean and free of disease, and both could be comfortable that they were protected from transmission of germs. I remember thinking how butchers began wearing white coats years before for simpler reasons—to keep their day clothes free of the stains of their occupation. Today, as I see patients—for diabetes, hypertension, gonorrhea, heart disease, high cholesterol, drug abuse, alcohol use, depression, and other medical problems— only a few will have contagious diseases, yet I still take refuge in my white coat.

Another reason physicians wear white coats is that patients expect us to wear white coats. The white coat adds the power of ritual to the strength of medical knowledge and skill, much the same way certain amulets and beads enhanced the powers of Indian shamans. The white coat helps develop the patient's confidence in the physician and helps form a trusting patient-physician relationship.

I remove a thread dangling from my coat sleeve. I wonder if another reason physicians wear white coats is because the coat still serves, in a vestigial way, its original function of protection, but now from emotions more than from germs. As physicians we no longer play the role of the country doctor who drives five miles on a snowy night to sit at the bedside of a feverish patient he has known for twenty years, providing that patient with reassurance, comfort, and what small amount of treatment there is to offer. Instead we often act as agents of technology and science, providing powerful treatments but little emotional support, to individuals overwhelmed by disease. I wonder whether we use our white coats to distance ourselves from our patients, to protect ourselves from sharing too intimately in our patient's pain, because the experience of disease is truly overwhelming and we feel fragile too. We accept this distance because we feel we have given the patient what he or she has come to us for, once we have given what technology has to offer.

I turn from the window and look down the hall at the four charts in the bin. I have a dull burning in the pit of my stomach. I straighten my white coat. There are patients to be seen. On days like today I doubt I could function without something to put on between me and my patients' pain.

Mr. Hurley is sitting in the next examination room. I say hello and he smiles as he struggles to right himself in the chair. He mumbles hello. He is a large man who is missing most of his teeth. His skin is pockmarked, he is wearing about eight layers of clothing, and he is sitting with a blank smile on his face as his head sways back and forth.

"What can we do for you today, Mr. Hurley?" I ask.

"I don't know," he says. I straighten out my white coat.

"Are you here to get your blood pressure checked?" I ask. He has hypertension and at his last visit, two months ago, we had increased the dose of his blood pressure medicines.

"Yeah. That must be it," he replies.

I notice a brown paper bag resting against the back leg of his chair. The bag is small and almost certainly contains a bottle of whiskey, which explains Mr. Hurley's slurred speech and difficulty sitting straight in his chair. We have talked about his drinking many times. I am not in the mood to discuss it again today.

"Have you been taking your medicines, Mr. Hurley?" I ask.

"Uh, no. Not lately. Not lately, now," he tells me, swaying to his right, and then regaining his balance.

"Were you taking them at all?" I ask. I am not sure why I am asking these questions. I know the answers, and each answer just frustrates me more.

"No, I ain't been taking the medicines all the time. I do take them sometimes, though, you know."

"Yeah," I say. I wrap the blood pressure cuff around his arm and pump up the bladder. While I'm pumping, Mr. Hurley, who is watching everything I do intently, belches in my face. The odor, a combination of alcohol and vomit, makes me nauseated. I turn my head away from him and lean back from what I am doing. Meanwhile, Mr. Hurley starts laughing his toothless laugh.

"I'm shorry, Doc," he says in a slurred voice,"I did'n know it uz coming out." He starts laughing again, trying not to.

I finish taking his blood pressure.

"Your blood pressure is fine today, Mr. Hurley. I don't know why, but your blood pressure is fine." I look at him and he reminds me of a hippopotamus in the zoo, grotesque and distorted, with two big teeth sticking out of his smile, but somehow likeable.

"I don't know whys either, Doc. I don't know why either."

I pick up the second chart from the pile in the bin. I am still thinking about Mr. Hurley. Why does he come in to the office? He doesn't take the medicines that I prescribe. He may not even need them anyway—he hasn't taken his medicine in months and his blood pressure was fine today. Yet at other visits, his blood pressure has been dangerously elevated. I don't have a good explanation for this. I open the next chart, Tamia Waverly's. She is a new patient to our office, twenty-two years old, and had been seen by one of the residents in the emergency room over the weekend for abdominal pain and nausea.

I walk down the hall to the examination room, open the door, and introduce myself. Tamia Waverly is a thin woman who has a strong, bony grip when we shake hands. She is wearing a blue T-shirt and a red cloth coat that is far too large for her. Her eyes are bloodshot with a yellow tinge and she has razor-thin eyebrows that slant in straight lines toward her ears. There is a large scar across her right cheek and another across her forehead. Her hair is pulled back in a red bandanna, her lips are thin and cracked, and the muscles of her neck look like thin strings. Her four-year-old daughter, standing next to her, smiles timidly then turns away from me and wraps her arms around her mother's leg.

"How are you feeling?" I ask.

"A little better. I don't got as bad belly pain right now and I'm not as nauseous. You know I was seen over the weekend, in the emergency room? Doctor says I got the yellow jaundice," she says.

"Yeah, I heard about that. The doctor you saw told me about you. He said you would be coming in."

"I'm still feeling nauseous, and I ain't eating much. But I'm feeling better than I was last week. What's this from, anyway?"

"It looks like you have hepatitis, which is an infection

of your liver. The blood tests that were drawn over the weekend showed that your liver is infected with hepatitis B. The virus that you have, hepatitis B, gets into your blood stream and . . ."

"A virus!" Her pupils grow wide. She reaches with her left hand and hugs her daughter's head into her thigh. "Hepatitis B, that's B for *bad*, right? I heard of that. Why I got it, and what's it doing to my body?"

"Hepatitis B is an infection of the liver that causes nausea and belly pain, like you were having." I can feel myself beginning to withdraw from her as she becomes upset. Taking refuge within my white coat, I focus on the clinical situation, rather than on Tamia's experience of disease, and on what the information means *to her*. If this were any other situation she would sense my withdrawal and resent it, but I am her doctor. My white coat grants me the authority to distance myself from her and still be accepted as a caring person. I continue, "You get hepatitis B from someone who already has it, either by having sex with them, by sharing a needle, or by a blood transfusion. If we can, we should try to figure out how you got the infection." I pause. She is sitting silently across from me, staring at the wall. "Are you sexually active?"

"I have sex, but not in a while."

"You shoot up?" I ask.

"Yeah, but I ain't done the needle in a long time. Lately I been doing the pipe. Even when I was using the needle, I was using clean needles, or I wash them with ammonia if I couldn't get no clean needles." By the pipe she means smoking crack cocaine, instead of injecting cocaine directly into her veins.

"When was the last time you shot up?" I ask her. Her daughter is rubbing her face along her mother's thigh and hugging her mother's leg with both hands.

"It been a while. I ain't done no needle in six months," Tamia replies.

"Have you had sex with anyone who might be shooting up?" I ask.

She bites her lower lip and turns her head to the side. Her face looks strained. "Could be," she says. "I been turning tricks on the streets for the last few months. You know, to make money for crack . . ."

She goes on to tell me that her cocaine habit was costing her two hundred dollars a day and that prostitution was the only way she could support it. She hasn't turned a trick in three weeks, though, she says. Then she lifts her daughter up into her lap, hugs her, and tells me that she loves her little girl, that her daughter has no one in the world to depend on but her, and that she is going to clean herself up.

"You think I got this hepatitis from turning tricks?" she asks.

"Probably, either from tricks or from a needle you used six months ago. . . ." I hesitate. I can feel the muscles in my face tighten as I try to find correct words to explain my next thought.

"What?" she asks, looking at me with large eyes.

"You got hepatitis from a needle or from sex. You can get AIDS the same way. Since you have hepatitis, we should check a blood test to see if you were also infected with the AIDS virus," I tell her.

"AIDS!?" She looks quickly at her daughter. Her mouth gapes. "What do you mean? You think I got AIDS? I can't have AIDS. I gotta . . . I gotta take care of Shaketa. Wha . . . where'd I get that from? Wha . . . what you talking 'bout?"

"I don't know if you have AIDS, but since you have hepatitis B it means you could have contracted AIDS as well. You may not have AIDS, but we don't know that. The only way we can know is by checking a blood test," I reply, holding back my emotions.

Tamia tucks her daughter's head into the nape of her neck and starts crying. A stream of tears falls to her daughter's hair. Shaketa is sitting quietly on her mother's lap, her nose twitching. I straighten out my white coat. I know I have other patients waiting to be seen, so I explain the AIDS blood test to Tamia while she is crying. I ask her to sign a consent form to have the test done. Then I get up, ask her to return in one week for the result, and leave the room.

Again there are four charts in the rack, four patients waiting in examination rooms. I am already tired and drained although it is only three o'clock. It is hard to keep up the vigilance I need here on days when I am feeling less than one hundred percent right myself. When I feel the way I do today it is difficult to be understanding to individuals who need it, who get understanding in few other places. Tania Waverly might have benefited from my staying to counsel her more, or simply from my being in the room with her while she cried, but today I leave the room when I'm done. The white coat reminds patients that the doctor is busy, and that most discussions need to fit into a twenty-minute time slot.

I take the top chart off the rack and begin reviewing it. It is May Haily's chart. She first came to our office three months ago because she was swollen across the right side of her face. It turned out that the man she was living with had hit her with the bottom of a crystal ashtray, breaking her jaw. It took a while for her to tell me that; she was embarrassed about having been treated that way. At that visit, and the next, we discussed her going for counseling at an organization, Women Against Abuse, that provides support and advice for women who have been beaten by husbands or boyfriends. I am not sure if she ever went for counseling. She did not return to the office for three months, then last week she came in because she had missed a period and was having profuse vaginal bleeding. On physical examination it looked as if she was spontaneously aborting a six-week pregnancy. I ordered laboratory tests and arranged follow-up to confirm that it was a miscarriage and not an ectopic pregnancy. We didn't have the time at that visit to talk about how things were going in her personal life. All I could gather from our short conversation was that she and her boyfriend had gotten back together and that now she was pregnant because he doesn't like using birth control.

Today she is here for a follow-up visit for her miscarriage, to make sure that the bleeding has stopped and that she has not developed fever or pain. Walking down the hall to her examination room, I notice her seven-year-old daughter standing outside the room. I smile at the girl, who seems uncomfortable but smiles back. When I walk through the doorway all I see is the green down vest of a middle-aged man leaning over and pressing against May Haily while she is sitting in her chair. He has his hand up her shirt, is giving her a big, open-mouthed kiss, and is pressing his leg between hers. I knock on the open door. Nothing. It doesn't interrupt the action for a second. I knock again. He turns around, feigns embarrassment, mumbles something that sounds like, "You know how it is," winks, and walks out of the room. Then he takes the seven-year-old's hand, and walks down the hall.

I stand in the room and look at May. She is looking at the ground and shaking her head. Dressed in a faded plaid flannel shirt and a denim skirt, she looks tired, and has dark circles under her eyes. Her hair is a soft black, flowing to her shoulders and curling under toward her collar like the bonnet of Michelangelo's *Pieta*. She has smooth skin and well-angled features. I ask her how she has been feeling since last week, not mentioning the way her boyfriend has just acted. She doesn't answer me; she just sits shaking her head and looking down at the ground. "What's the matter?" I ask. She continues shaking her head, looks up for a second, then looks back down. She begins rubbing her hands up and down the fabric of her skirt. "What's the matter?" I repeat.

Still staring into her lap, she starts, "Na . . . nothing. I got a lot a things on my mind. A lot going on."

"Anything you want to talk about?" I ask, though I know I don't feel like talking today. In addition, I am hesitant to probe too much. I don't want to alienate her, and I am not sure how much of this is my business.

"No. I just got some thinking to do, a lot of thinking to do."

"Thinking about what?" I ask. Again, I am not sure if this is a door I want to open. I have other patients waiting, I'm already behind schedule, and I'm not sure I will have much to offer her if she does choose to confide in me.

"Just thinking. Thinking."

"Have you had further bleeding since last week?" I ask, changing the subject.

"No, no more bleeding," she replies in a quivering voice. She takes a deep breath, lets it out, and begins shaking her head again. Her whole body begins trembling.

"He . . . You . . . you told me not to have sex this week . . . while I was bleeding. . . . He . . . he made me have sex with him . . . tw . . . twice. . . . I didn't want to, I didn't really want to," she says, her eyes red and filling with tears.

"He forced you to have sex?" I ask. I cringe as the words come out of my mouth. Why can't I find words that are more understanding and sympathetic? I sound like a defense attorney cross-examining a witness.

"He didn't force me . . . but I didn't really want to, you know."

"Has he hit you again in the last few months?"

"Oh, he hit me a few times, you know, and I don't like that. Nothing like when he hit me before."

"Do you plan to do anything about that?" I ask. My words are not coming out right. They sound accusatory. I know I'm not handling this situation as well as I would like to. I believe that somehow, what I say to her, if I choose the right words, may help her. Only I can't seem to find the right words. I wish there were someone to turn to for advice, as there was in medical school, where there was always an attending physician with a great deal of experience—or at least one who acted as if he had a great deal of experience. Now I am the attending physician. I have been for almost a year and a half. I feel as if there is something more I could be doing for her, but I don't know what. If May Haily were a child I would put her in the hospital to protect her from her home environment, but she is not a child and so she has to make her own choices.

I repeat, "Is there anything you plan to do about your situation?"

"I don't know," she replies. "I been thinking about it. I'll see. . . . I'll . . ." Her voice drifts off.

"It's an awful situation," I respond, shaking my head. I notice a loose thread hanging from a button of my white coat and pull the thread off. I'm angry. I'm angry at him for treating her this way. I'm angry at her for staying with him and putting up with this type of treatment. I'm also angry with myself because I feel helpless. I am trying, but I can't think of anything to do or say that will help her.

"Do you think that living with him is the best idea for you?" I ask. I try to let her come to her own conclusion. She doesn't. We discuss her situation further. Her boyfriend often acts inappropriately in public places, like the way he was trying to make out with her when I walked into the exam room. I ask May, as I did three months ago, if she has thought of enrolling for counseling with Women Against Abuse. I ask her if she has thought of anything else she might do to change her predicament with her boyfriend.

She tells me that she has thought about counseling but hasn't done anything about it. She has also thought about leaving her boyfriend, and maybe will someday, but the last time she was going to leave he held a knife to her neck, while her daughter was in the room, and threatened to slit her throat if she walked out the door. Besides, he has guns in the house, which he said he would use to come after her if she snuck away, and she really isn't sure that she wants to sneak away anyway.

We continue to talk. Mostly I listen. She tells me about a world that is very different from the one I know. I grew up in a middle-class suburb of New York City, where rules were often bent or broken, but where it was usually clear to me that rules existed and what those rules were. She is from the inner city. Her world is harder and tougher than mine. The rules, which must exist, are often not clear to me. I have no idea of the parameters of behavior in her world—what is tolerated, what is considered the norm. Not knowing the territory, how can I advise her as my patient? It is easy to say she should leave him, but where would she go? And can she leave him if he is putting a knife to her throat, and she still loves him?

It is now four o'clock. In the last hour I have seen a middle-aged man with a sore throat, an older woman with a respiratory infection, and a fifteen-year-old with a cold who needed a doctor's note for school. The next two patients are infants who have been brought in by their mothers for well-baby exams and immunizations. Both infants are growing well and both women seem to be holding up under the pressures of being new mothers. Both are receiving a good deal of help from their families. Tanya, the younger of the two, has returned to school and hopes to finish tenth grade in the spring. That takes a lot of work, and so far she is doing it. I see a two-year-old boy I've taken care of since birth. He is now running about the room climbing on chairs and playing with a toy space ship. I talk with his mother and examine him. It is a pleasure to see that he is growing well with the nurturing of a supportive family.

The last patient of the day is Mya Jones. Mya is thirty-four years old and comes to the office about once every four months when she is feeling more depressed than usual and wants someone to talk to. Sitting in the examination room with Mya always makes me feel uncomfortable. She has dyed blonde hair, wears tight pants and close-fitting shirts, and always tries to make more eye contact with me than I am comfortable with.

I stand outside her room and make sure my white coat is completely buttoned. I open her chart and see that she has not come in for a single scheduled appointment in two years. Every office visit has been for an acute crisis, usually revolving around her deepening depression over a boyfriend that has left her. We have referred her for psychological counseling a number of times but she has never kept these appointments. I am not sure she receives any benefit from her visits to our office. Whatever is wrong when she walks into the office is just as wrong when she leaves. Yet she returns, and today she may be suicidal, or have an infection, and so must be seen.

I walk into the room, say hello, and sit in a chair about five feet from her. I ask her what is wrong today and she tells me that she is depressed, has been doing a large amount of cocaine, and is now coming down from her high because her supply ran out. She would like to be admitted to a drug rehabilitation center. This is the first time that I have heard Mya take initiative to ask for something that may help her. Though I feel her chances of following through with the program are small, she is at least making an effort, and I feel I should be supportive of it.

I spend half an hour talking with Mya about drug rehabilitation. Then I leave the exam room and walk down the hall to the nurses' station to phone the rehabilitation center and request that Mya be admitted. The receptionist at the rehabilitation center takes Mya's information and puts me on hold for about five minutes. When she gets back on the line she tells me that because Mya lives in District 1 the admission will have to be arranged through a different facility. Over the next fifteen minutes and two more phone calls, I find out that the correct rehabilitation center is closed to admissions the rest of the day, but that an admission can be arranged for late tomorrow morning. While making the phone calls I am thinking that this is a lot of time and effort to be taking for someone who is probably going to score some cocaine tonight and not even consider going to the rehabilitation center tomorrow. The cynicism I feel toward Mya bothers me. I was not this wary of patients a year ago, when I first started to work in this office. I am not sure whether I am becoming too hardened and cynical, or whether I am simply beginning to acknowledge some difficult truths.

I ask the nurse to finish making the arrangements for the rehabilitation admission and to explain to Mya what she will need to do, then I go back to my consultation room. I lean against my desk and stare out the window toward the vacant lot across the street. The beam the boy was walking on sits across the two cinder blocks. At the corner of the lot closest to the church two men are talking to one another. I watch as they exchange money and a small bag, then walk off in opposite directions. An old woman wearing a thick gray sweater walks slowly and carefully on the sidewalk in front of the church, carrying a plastic bag filled with groceries. A young child wearing a blue zip-up coat is sitting on the third step of a boarded-up brick building next to the church, throwing rocks at a fire hydrant. An orange glow in the sky creates the illusion for a moment that the church is on fire.

I take off my white coat and hang it on the hook behind the door. It is dirty around the cuffs. There is a small blue mark by the right hip pocket from Gram's solution that splattered as I prepared a sputum specimen for viewing under the microscope. The coat has protected my clothes, but it has not protected me from my patients' pain. At the end of the week I will send the coat to the cleaners; when it returns, pressed and clean, the lives of the patients I have seen today will have changed little. Each day I feel my patients' sense of frustration and futility more deeply. At the end of each day, even sometimes—like today—at the beginning, I feel helpless and overwhelmed. Not by the medical problems I see—some are challenging, some are not. Rather, I now understand and share my patients' sense that the problems they face daily may be too large to fight against.

I turn, open the briefcase on my desk, place my stethoscope and reflex hammer inside, then click the briefcase closed. I am being changed here. I am becoming hardened. Slowly. I can feel it in the words that come out as I talk to patients. I can sense it in certain attitudes when I walk into patients' rooms. I am not sure how much longer I can provide medical care in this setting before I lose the compassion for patients that is essential if I am to continue to practice medicine. I pick up my briefcase. It is time to go home. I will be back tomorrow.

Icarus

THROUGH THE IRON-FRAMED windows I can see the sun setting over the tall buildings. It is early March, the air is damp and cold. The monthly administrative meeting for the department that runs the office has been going on for about forty-five minutes in a conference room on the eighth floor of the university building. The room is lined with oak shelves, and the shelves are filled with medical books and journals. Twelve physicians, including myself, each wearing a white coat or a sports coat and a tie, are sitting around a large oak table. There is a typed agenda on the table in front of each physician.

"As some of you know, . . ." The chairman hesitates before beginning the seventh item on the agenda. "Some of our offices have been severely affected by funding cuts on federal, state, and local levels that have affected reimbursement of medical care for the urban poor. . . ." He re-arranges the papers in front of him, then continues. "Some offices are not even meeting overhead expenses, and have been operating at a considerable loss. In order to continue providing care at other sites, we will be closing the southern neighborhood office on July the first."

I was told before the meeting that the office would be

closing, but hearing the chairman's announcement brings home the reality of the decision. I think of little Ezekiel and his mother. Where will they go for their medical care? My mind wanders to May Haily and Ralph Gregory. Will they make even the small effort required to obtain medical care elsewhere?

I look out the window. The lights in the office buildings across the street flicker like fireflies at dusk. The muscles in my face tense. I strain to see in the lights some glimmer of hope, to recognize in the beauty that exists within the city's decay some sense of purpose or meaning. I think of Ezekiel, who continues to gain weight and develop as he should for his age. I think of Ezekiel's father, who wants better for his children than he has had for himself, and of the strength he has displayed by overcoming his drug addiction and staying clean. I think of the way he has taken advantage of the help available to him through a local drug rehabilitation program. I think of Marjeta Bradley, who returned to our office one month ago dressed in a beige suit and hat. At first I didn't recognize her. I hadn't seen her in the year since her ectopic pregnancy. During that year she had enrolled in a rehabilitation program, with the help of which she stopped using drugs; then she began working as a receptionist. Now, with the help of her mother, she is taking good care of her six-year-old daughter, Tamia. Ms. Bradley returned to our office for routine health care, a pap smear, and a prescription for birth control pills. If I had to have guessed a year ago, I would have thought she might not be alive by now. I think of Patricia Doughty, who came into the office six months ago because she was concerned that she had lost twenty pounds. She was having trouble sleeping at night, felt washed out, and was worried that she had AIDS. She didn't have AIDS, but she was depressed, a feeling that began after her most recent boyfriend had left her. We treated her with an antidepressant and supportive counseling and she began to feel better over the next few weeks. In the next three months she gained back all the weight she had lost and started going back to work.

I have witnessed individuals in this neighborhood demonstrate their capacity to put their lives back together after the most difficult of situations: strong drug addictions, family members shot and killed, abuse by spouses or parents. I have seen them find meaning in their lives. One woman I take care of has brought up fifty-eight foster children over the last thirty years. She is sixty years old and currently has six children in her home. She is a religious woman and she feels that she owes this to her people, and to God. She also loves children. I have seen deep reservoirs of strength in my patients, but they and their families fight daily against an unhealthy, dangerous environment and they need help in order to tap these strengths. I have worked with individuals who have had dreams, who have hoped to change their lives, and have succeeded in overcoming the difficulties that surrounded them; I have seen individuals who have no dreams, or who have broken dreams, or dreams that have dried up and wilted, who may never change their lives. I have learned that hope, without help, withers and dies. As funds for medical care in the inner city continue to diminish, as social programs become more scarce, as medical offices like ours are forced to close, people who have the greatest number of problems will have fewer and fewer places to turn for help.

I look around the room. Across from me one physician is writing a note on a yellow pad of paper. Two physicians at the far end of the table are whispering to each other and one smiles. Around the table others are listening to the chairman, or looking down. I wonder what they are thinking. I have known most of them for years, and they are all dedicated, bright, caring people. Yet none of them has indicated any concerns that the office is closing. Is this decision bothering any of them? I look down at the table. The grain of the light polished oak flows in swirls around the typed sheet of tonight's agenda. The chairman's voice seems to fade as he begins the next item.

I shut my eyes, feeling off balance, and I see a man falling, tumbling, from the sky. W. H. Auden's poem, "Musée des Beaux Arts," describes a painting by the Danish master, Pieter Brueghel. In that painting, Icarus, the mythological character who flew too close to the sun in wings formed from wax and feathers, is depicted at the end of his fall, after his wings have melted, a moment before he is engulfed by the sea. In the forefront of the painting a plowman is casually plowing his fields. In the background a beautiful ship is moving on with billowing sails. Icarus, for whom the painting is named, is barely visible. If you look carefully you can see two pale legs sticking out of the green sea. Auden describes the scene:

> . . . how everything turns away
> Quite leisurely from the disaster; the ploughman may
> Have heard the splash, the forsaken cry,
> But for him it was not an important failure; . . .
> . . . and the expensive delicate ship that must have seen

Something amazing, a boy falling out of the sky,
Had somewhere to get to and sailed calmly on.

I open my eyes. The closing of our office represents an important failure—for myself, those around me, and our government—and I watch myself join my colleagues' silence. I am sure our office is not the only family medicine office in the country that is shutting its doors. As a society we have found the resources to fund research into cures for rare diseases but we have not discovered within ourselves a reason to use the knowledge we have to help hundreds of thousands of men, women, and children who live within blocks of our largest research centers.

I look past the wrought-iron bars of the window. The orange glow of the setting sun appears to set the city aflame. I think of Watts in the late 1960s, south central Los Angeles in the 1990s. The frustrations, disappointments, angers, resentments, the physical and psychological pains that my patients carry with them when they walk into my office, their lack of concern for their own bodies, their feeling that they have little to lose are many of the same feelings that lead to the burning of our cities. Over the last few years small outbreaks of violence have occurred in almost every major metropolitan area in the United States. In September 1988, I was walking down the street in Philadelphia when a rowdy crowd started gathering. I didn't like the feel of things so I got in my car and drove across the Ben Franklin Bridge. The next day I read in the paper that hundreds of youths had taken to South Street after a concert, smashing store windows and beating up bystanders. In Chicago, July 1990, within minutes after a generating plant left the east side of the city without electricity, people began looting stores, smashing windows and walls. In May 1991, in Washington D.C., for two straight nights, cars were set on fire, stores were looted, and general rioting took place that caused more than $2 million in damages. Outbursts of random group violence have become commonplace, like brush fires in a dry forest, the spontaneous igniting of a destructive force in a susceptible environment. Most of these events go unnoticed as they are reported in small columns tucked into the middle pages of newspapers.

I think back three months ago, to early January, when I met with the chairman and explained that I had decided I would leave the office this coming July. He listened carefully as I described my frustration with seeing patients who had overwhelming social and medical problems that they often did not seem to want to address, and my frustration at working in an environment that did not have sufficient social services to assist me in helping my patients. I told him how, over time, I began to feel closer to my patients and was able to see the social gulfs that separated us being bridged, and how I began to appreciate and like my patients as individuals. Then, after a while, I found myself withdrawing from patients, becoming calloused to their problems and needs, in order to protect myself from their pain. The chairman listened carefully. I assumed that he would find someone to work in the office after I left. He did not. If I could not continue working there, what right did I have to expect another person to take my place?

I look around the table. I want to try to convince the people sitting around this table that we should keep the office open. I would like to offer to stay on and continue to provide medical care in the office. Yet I hold back. My experience has changed me—as a person and as a physician. I realize that continuing to work in our neighborhood office would require personal sacrifices greater than I am willing to make.

There is a bustle of movement. The people around the table are gathering their papers and getting up from their chairs. As I stand, frustration rises within me. I realize there is nothing I can do to change the fact that in three months our office will close—or that there is nothing I want to do.

Spring

I PARK MY CAR half a block from the office and step out into the cool morning air. The street is quiet and the sun is just beginning to peek over the brick buildings. I take a deep breath, then open my trunk to get my briefcase and stethoscope.

"Hi, Doctor," I hear someone call from behind me. I turn and see Taneta Bradley walking toward me, carrying a little baby strapped like a papoose across her chest. I last saw Taneta in the office about eight months ago. "You seen my baby yet?" she asks me.

"No. I'd love to," I reply. My mind wanders back, almost a year, to when I told Taneta that she was pregnant and she sat crying in my office. I saw her three times that week as we discussed her feelings about whether or not she wanted to have an abortion.

Taneta crosses the street. She is wearing a light blue T-shirt, with Southside Junior High written in bright yellow letters across the front. She told me during one of her office visits that she won that shirt last year when she was voted the most valuable player in her seventh-grade basketball league. When she wore that shirt she walked with pride, and now she was walking with pride carrying her baby across the street.

"What do you think, Doctor?" she tilts her head and smiles at me. Her baby is dressed in a pink frilly dress and a bonnet with white lace. Its head is lying quietly across Taneta's left breast. Her smile is beaming as she looks back down at her little girl. A feeling of promise and hope seems to flutter between her and the baby as the sun is rising above the tenement buildings.

"She's beautiful," I say, taking a deep breath of the fresh morning air. "What's her name?"

"Lucy," she replies, and smiles at me.

"How are you doing?" I ask.

"Good," she says, her voice like a song.

"Are you still going to school?"

"Yeah," she says, then pauses. "I'm going to summer school so I can finish eighth grade. If I go all summer they said they'd let me graduate."

"That's good. It's important that you take care of yourself as well as take care of the baby." I smile at her. "Is your boyfriend still with you?"

"No, he and me broke up two months ago, but I got a new one now. He's nice." Taneta's eyes drop shyly to the ground.

"Are you using birth control?" I ask. A little over a year ago I had seen Taneta in the office every other week for two or three months, hoping that frequent visits would allow me to address any side effects she might be having from the birth control pills and that the visits would help to reinforce the importance of taking her pills.

"Nah. They gave them to me in the hospital. But I just

haven't been taking them. I'm not going to get pregnant now, I just had a baby. I can never remember to take them pills anyhow," Taneta replies. She looks at her baby, then smiles. "I got a lot to take care of now, you know. See ya."

She turns and walks away with a spring in her step. I turn and walk across the street to the office.

You Know Me
Better Than Anyone

IT HAS BEEN two weeks since the chairman's announcement that our office will be closing. It is eleven o'clock in the morning and I stand again looking out the consultation room window. The rain has ended and water fills the ruts and cracks of the street and sidewalk. The sun is reflecting in rainbow colors off the windows of the project building one block away. Four older men, each carrying a metal folding chair, step out from the side of the large building, walk across the courtyard, and set their chairs against a fence. Two young children are kicking a ball twenty feet from where the men sit; an old lady walks across the courtyard carrying an empty shopping bag in one hand and a cane in the other.

I turn, sit down at my desk, and pick up the first lab report from a stack piled on the corner of my desk. The test results are from blood we drew three days ago on Ameta Barnett, a cute three-year-old who was in the office three days ago for a routine check-up. Her test shows that she has large amounts of lead in her blood. This probably comes from her eating or chewing chips of lead-based paint that is peeling off the walls of the old apartment building she lives in. An elevated level of lead in a child's blood can impair the development of the nervous system, leading to lower IQ, problems with coordination, and even seizures. Ideally, the health department would look into the source of Ameta's lead exposure and take steps to correct it. Unfortunately, they too are underfunded, and I have heard various reports about how well they are actually able to carry out their work. My next step will be to draw another lab test to confirm the high lead level and to see whether Ameta will need medication to remove lead from her body. I pick up the phone and call Ameta's mother. A recording indicates that the number is disconnected, so I dictate a letter hoping they still live at the address listed on the chart.

The next report confirms a diagnosis of gonorrhea in a woman I treated for a pelvic infection four days ago. I glance through her chart and see that this is her third episode of gonorrhea in the last two years. I make a note in her chart so that if she comes back for her scheduled follow-up appointment, I will discuss with her her risk for AIDS.

I look back out the window. The courtyard next to the projects is busy. A group of teenagers are playing basketball at its far end. A bright red Cadillac with gold trim and whitewall tires is parked on the corner, outside the fence, and a group of men and women are talking to the driver. Children are running and pushing at each other on the sidewalk. Later today our practice administrators, our nurse, our receptionist, and I will meet for the first time to begin working out the logistics involved in closing the office. We will need to decide when to start telling patients that the office is closing, whom to refer our patients to, where patients' medical charts will be stored, when the phone system should be shut off, and all the other details we can think of. I am filled with sadness. I begin to realize the degree to which this office has become part of my life. I am already mourning the severing of relationships with patients who I have come to know and tried to understand.

I step back from the window and notice a ray of light that lands on the shelves of the far wall, illuminating textbooks of pediatrics, internal medicine, family medicine, gynecology, and pharmacology. When I first arrived at this office almost two years ago, fresh out of residency, I thought I would be practicing family medicine with a challenging patient population. I could not have predicted the depth of human encounters; nor could I have imagined the sadness I would feel today upon preparing to leave. My medicine has allowed me to touch the lives of people I would otherwise probably never have met, and it has allowed their lives to touch mine. For the last two years I have felt like a traveler in a foreign country, watching with wide eyes the people and their customs, all the time working only a fifteen-minute walk from the apartment where I have lived for five years. I have witnessed things beautiful, terrible, and mundane in a medical practice that has not accomplished anything remarkable, but at least has succeeded in doing something ordinary—providing high-quality medical care in a respectful and caring manner—in a neighborhood where so little that is ordinary ever occurs.

Janet, the nurse, knocks on the door and tells me that a radiologist is on the phone. He wants to discuss a chest x-ray of a patient we sent to the hospital this morning. The patient is twenty-seven years old and he came to the office with mild but progressive shortness of breath. The radiologist tells me that the chest x-ray shows an "interstitial" pneumonia, most likely pneumocystis pneumonia, which is the most common way that AIDS begins. I decide to send the patient, who is still in the x-ray department, to the emergency room where one of my associates will meet him, discuss his diagnosis with him, and then admit him to the hospital.

I hang up the phone and walk back to the window. Outside, the sun is still shining. Children are still playing kickball in the courtyard. As I think about the patients I have cared for over the last two years, I realize that part of my frustration comes from dwelling on cases where my best efforts have been thwarted.

During the last two years I have often thought about Taneta Avery, a sixty-year-old woman who walked into the office because she had an uncomfortable feeling in her belly. When I examined her I felt a mass over her liver. The ultrasound scan I ordered showed she had a tumor. She did not return to the office to discuss the results of her scan, as I had asked her to do. Over the next two months I tried calling her and wrote her numerous letters, emphasizing how important it was to come back to the office so that we could arrange treatment for her condition. She never returned.

Salema Reed was a thin woman who came into our office because she had been losing weight and running high fevers for three months. Her chest x-ray, performed a mile from our office at the hospital's radiology department, showed a fulminant tuberculosis infection. She was supposed to return to our office that afternoon to go over the results and plan for treatment of her infection. She never came back. Since there was no phone number on her chart, I dictated a letter to her. I sent the letter by certified mail, return receipt requested, since I was also concerned that I might be held liable for failure to follow up and treat her infection. I contacted the public health department, thinking of the other people that she might infect. The certified letter came back to the office with "No Such Address" stamped in red across the front. I checked to make sure that the address on the letter was filled out correctly, then asked the police to try to contact her at home. They personally visited the address on our chart and found that it was a demolished building.

I am haunted by thoughts of these individuals, and others. One night, shopping in the supermarket, I squeezed a small melon to see if it was ripe. The melon was the same size and shape as the mass I had felt in Ms. Avery's abdomen. I wondered if her tumor had spread, if she was in pain, if she was still alive. Although I know that I am not responsible for her failure to return to the office, I was involved in her care, and periodically I think of her and feel for the pain she might be in.

One night, on my way to see a theater production, I walked past a woman who was lying on the sidewalk wrapped in a blanket. Her face was dirty, she was thin, and she had long, stringy black hair. Our eyes met briefly, then she started coughing, spit thick mucous onto the sidewalk, and pulled the blanket over her head. I thought of Salema Reed, and I wondered how many people she had infected with tuberculosis since she first came coughing into our office. Half a block later I turned around and all I could see was the outline of a large brown blanket that moved slightly with the sound of each fading cough.

I sometimes think about the twenty-seven-year-old man who came into the office to be tested for HIV. He had used

IV drugs in the past. He came because one of his close friends had been diagnosed as having AIDS. We talked for a long time before drawing his blood. He never returned to our office for the test results. The blood test indicated that he was infected with HIV. I think about the young, blind woman who came into the office carrying a bible, able to recite passages from memory. She was living on the street, she told me, and she was having headaches and trouble hearing out of her left ear. A careful examination and a CAT scan showed that she had a tumor on the left side of her brain. She walked out of the radiology department before we could admit her to the hospital, and so far has not come back to the office. We have no way of contacting her since she has no home, and treatment of her disease will have to wait until she one day wanders into our office, or another office, or an emergency room, because her headache has become intolerable, or because she has had a seizure, or because she can no longer hear or move an arm or a leg.

I do not think as much about patients whose treatment and follow-up care have gone smoothly, even though there are more of them than there are patients who don't return. Betty Carter is a woman who came in to our office with frequent one-sided headaches. I diagnosed her as having migraines, and prescribed the appropriate medication. She now comes in, without headaches, about every six months for a follow-up check. I seldom think about her at times other than her office visit. Nor do I think about the teenage girl who came in for birth control pills five months ago, whom I saw again a month later to check on side effects and to encourage to take her pills, and whom I have not seen since then because she has not become pregnant.

I often think about Ariel Jones, a fourteen-year-old girl who came to the office with a cold. While talking to her I also discovered that she was sexually active and not using birth control. I took the time to counsel her carefully, and pre-scribed birth control pills. She returned to the office three months later, pregnant, wanting an abortion. I don't think a great deal about Emma Townsend, a sixty-three-year-old woman who had a heart attack seven years ago, who I see every three months to check on her hypertension and her high cholesterol. She takes her medicines effortlessly, has excellent blood pressure and cholesterol control, and her office visits usually last about five minutes. I have the feel-ing that I am not doing anything for her, she is doing so well, but when I look back in her chart I see that I have changed her medicines three times in the last two years.

A car stops across the street from our office and a young man, about sixteen, helps an elderly woman from the car and up the steps of the apartment building on the far side of the vacant lot. Will my patients care that our office is closing? A few will. Particularly the older ones who have become used to our office and the way it operates, who have become used to their doctor, and for whom change is diffi-cult. There is Luceta Reagan, who was ninety-three years old this past May and who I have seen about once a month for the past two years, almost always with the same complaint, "I'm just not feeling right, I'm soooo tired." I've searched but I can't find anything wrong with her, except age, which is bound to make anyone a little tired. Yet, in spite of all her complaining when she sees me, she does her own shopping twice a week, cleans her own home, and makes sure she regularly sees her grandchildren, great-grandchildren, and the great-great-grandchildren who live down the block from her.

Irene Baker comes into the office once every three months to have her blood pressure checked. She has been on the same two medicines for fifteen years now, wears a clove of garlic around her neck, and refuses to have the medicines changed, even when her blood pressure is higher than it should be. I've explained to her many times that she should be on different medicine, that the medicine she is taking is probably not the best for her. "Doctor," she tells me, "I know what's good for me." And after two years of taking care of her, I am beginning to believe that she probably does.

An occasional younger patient will miss the office as well. Melvina King, a pretty sixteen-year-old girl, came to the office with her mother on Good Friday, feeling tired and thirsty. We diagnosed Melvina as having diabetes and we saw her in the office every day for the next two weeks, teaching her about diabetes and how to give herself shots of insulin. Now she controls her blood sugar perfectly, has an excellent knowledge of diabetes, and comes in to see us about every two to three months. She is looking forward to graduating from high school and plans to become a nurse.

The number of people who will miss our office is greater than I first thought it would be, and is probably even greater than I now believe. Two years ago, when I finished residency and moved from the larger main office where we trained as residents across town to this neighborhood office, I knew that certain patients would follow me. There were others I could not have guessed would make that effort. Donnette Hughs, a patient I took care of during the three years of my residency, is in her mid-sixties, obese, has hypertension, and suffers from arthritis in her knees. She lives with her sister in a small apartment on the other side of the city. For three years, during her office visits, I would suggest ways for her to try to lose weight and recommend changes in her medications. I always felt as though she was not hearing what I was saying as she sat on the exam table staring blankly back at me. One morning, a month after I had moved to this neighborhood office, I walked into an exam room and was surprised to see Ms. Hughs sitting on the examination table, just as she had been sitting every two months for the previous three years. When I shared with her my surprise, because I knew that coming to the new office meant she had to take an extra bus ride, she looked up at me with an shy smile and replied, "Of course I followed you, Doctor, you known me for three years, you know me better than anyone in the whole world."

Last Day

IT IS EARLY MORNING. The hallway of the office is illuminated by an exit sign above the fire escape door. The exam rooms on either side of the hallway are locked. I walk past the nurses' station and hear the hum of the refrigerator in which we store the vaccines. At the end of the hall, I unlock the consultation room door and walk in. My desk is neat for the first time in two years, and only a few lab results that require my attention remain in the box.

I place my briefcase on the desk and look out the window. Across the street a mother is walking with a young child past the lot where the Street Sound Bar used to be. Down the block the projects tower over the neighborhood. In half an hour we will open the doors to our office for the last time. We will see a few scheduled patients, a few unscheduled patients, and then, mid-afternoon, we will lock the doors and leave.

I sit at my desk, take the stethoscope from my briefcase, and place it in the pocket of my white coat. I will miss this office and the patients I have taken care of. I have learned a great deal here. I have learned how to tolerate frustration and still care about people; I have learned that there are different things that I can do for different people; I have learned that people I thought I barely knew sometimes feel I know them best; I have learned that the people I think I know I may know least. I have learned to trust my instincts, that I can make a diagnosis by the way a patient walks through the door; I have learned that my instincts can fool me, as can my physical exam, and lab tests, and x-rays, and that some synthesis of all that I know and all that I feel is sometimes correct and is sometimes incorrect but is all I can do. I have learned that caring goes further than cure because the cures are few and far between and caring shares its healing powers with every patient who walks through the door, leaving the door open for the patient to return. I have learned that deeds speak louder than words, but that words are often the most important tool we have when we are with a patient—those words are played over and over again for the patient, and the patient's friends and family, to hear; I have learned that words must be carefully chosen, honed and polished like fine tools that open secret locks. I have learned that all I can be is one person with one mind and one body and one set of hands, and that my hands will help some and not help others but that I must make sure I always have enough caring and energy to help at least myself. I have learned that there are limits to my knowledge, and I reach those limits daily; I have learned that when knowledge isn't the limit, other limits remain—my personality, my patients' personalities, patients' abilities to take medicines, patients' lifestyles, the environment we are all living in. I have learned that socio-cultural boundaries will exist, and add flavor to life, yet honesty, concern, and respect for the individual creates bridges that can allow me to communicate and touch another person over the chasms of life's differences. I have learned that I will learn from people and events that I don't plan on learning from more than from people and events I plan to learn from.

The elevator door at the end of the hall creaks open. I turn and take the small stack of lab tests from the box behind me. Janet knocks on the door and asks if I am ready for the day. I look up, and we hold each other's gaze for a few moments. I tell her I am ready and she nods. Then she smiles, turns, and walks down the hall; I can hear her unlocking the examination room doors.

The first patient of the day is Carlotta Mavery. Carlotta made an appointment yesterday because she has been having pain in the lower part of her belly. I know Carlotta's whole family, though I've only seen Carlotta herself a few times. Carlotta lives with her mother, six brothers and sisters, an elderly aunt, and her grandmother in a three-bedroom apartment two blocks from our office. Carlotta is a thin, shy, immature thirteen-year-old.

I walk into the exam room and say hello. Carlotta's eyes are focused on the sink. She is wearing a blue T-shirt with "Nick's Hardware" written in yellow italics across the front and she has on a red baseball cap. I ask her what brought her to the office today.

"I been having these pains across my belly," she says. Her right palm is resting against the middle of her abdomen. "I figured I'd come in and find out what they was."

"How long have you been having these pains?" I ask.

"Four or five months," she says.

"When do they seem to come on?"

"Usually late in the morning."

"Around what time?"

"Oh, around eleven o'clock."

"Are the pains worse on weekends?"

"No." She pauses and thinks for a minute. "No, they don't seem to come on the weekends."

We talk some more. Eleven o'clock is when she takes English class in her junior high school. Some of the boys in the class are rowdy and one in particular has been coming on to Carlotta. She is not interested, but doesn't really know how to handle the attention. She worries about the class all morning. In addition, there are often fights in the hallway in her school. After performing a physical exam, which is normal, I reassure Carlotta that there is nothing wrong with her body. We talk about social pressures and I support her decision not to go out with the boy if she does not want to. She is relieved, she tells me; she was worried that she had stomach cancer, which, she learned in health class, has become more common over the last twenty years.

Our next patient is Amelia Chase. Mrs. Chase is sixty-two years old and I have been taking care of her for five years, first in our main office, now in this one. I pick up her chart and see that Mrs. Chase is here for a "check-up." I walk in the room, extend my hand, and say hello.

"Put your hand back," she snaps, her head held high. "I am mad!" She is wearing a white lace dress and a white hat with a powder-blue ribbon around the brim. A mahogany cane is leaning on the wall next to her. Her upper lip is drawn tight over her teeth, she begins to rock her head back and forth, and then continues in her crisp Southern accent, "How you think you can just leave like that? I followed you over here, I've been riding extra buses, costing me an extra dollar twenty-five cents every time I come to see you. Now you are leaving, just when I am going to need you most, in my old age? You are my doctor, you can't just up and leave like that. Who do you think you are?"

I think back two years ago to when I took care of Mrs. Chase in the hospital when she was admitted for pneumonia. She almost died—she had to spend three days in the intensive care unit. Even in the hospital she maintained a sense of dignity and control. I think about the discussions we have had about whether she should have surgery on the vessels in her legs, which have been slowly closing to the point that she now develops pain after walking twenty feet. She does not want surgery, she has told me, because doctors "experiment on poor people." I have tried to explain to her that isn't the case, but she has her beliefs. I am different from other doctors, she has told me, because I talk to her and I understand her, but I am not that different, and she has not taken my recommendation for the pains in her legs.

I sit down across from her. She is looking at me expectantly. "I'm going to miss seeing you in the office," I say.

"I don't know why," she snaps. "You always just rushes into the room and rushes out, never doing anything for me. You doctors are some bunch, seeing people when they are in pain, then charging them money . . ." She pauses, shifts in her seat, clears her throat, then says, "We two sure did get along, didn't we? For a doctor and a patient, I mean. I mean, *especially* for a doctor and a *poor* patient. Oh, I'm sure you have your reasons for leaving, but don't you ever forget ol' Amelia, you hear. Wherever you go, you make sure always do stay in touch." Then she points her finger at me.

"You just sitting there like a bump on a log. You gonna listen to my heart today or just keep sitting there?"

I walk to her, stand on her right side, and lean over and place my stethoscope over the front of her dress. The cotton frill brushes my fingers as I listen to the regular rhythm of her heart. I move my stethoscope to her back and listen to the clear movement of air in and out of her lungs, then I lightly touch her shoulder. "Your heart and lungs sound good," I say. She looks up and nods.

I sit back down and pull out my prescription pad. "Make sure you keep taking your blood pressure medicines. Here is the name of a doctor you can use. I will send him a letter about you. He will take good care of you." I nod reassuringly and hand her the sheet of paper.

We look at each other, then rise from our chairs. She takes her cane from the wall, steadies herself, and begins to walk toward the door. As she walks past me she taps me twice, playfully, on my leg with her cane. Then she takes a step without the cane, starts to lose her balance, and begins to teeter, her arms out and cane in the air. I reach toward her and she puts her arms around me, pulling me close. I feel the fabric of her dress, and her small, frail body against mine as we embrace.

The rest of the morning is quiet. A few scheduled patients come in for a last check of their hypertension or diabetes. We are done with the morning by eleven-thirty and I go down the block to pick up lunch for myself, the receptionist, and the nurse. In twenty minutes I return with pizza.

We eat in the consultation room. Janet will start work next week in an inpatient department of the hospital. She is looking forward to new challenges and a more controlled environment. Loreene, the receptionist, will work as a receptionist in another department of the hospital. As for myself, I am looking for a practice outside of the city.

The afternoon is slow. We have not scheduled any patients, so we have time to clean up the office and gather our belongings. Over the course of the afternoon I see a couple of children with stuffed noses and sore throats. At three-thirty I see a woman who has been running a fever of 103° and who appears to have a pelvic infection. I give her a shot of antibiotics and arrange a follow-up appointment for her at our other office, a little over a mile away.

I walk back down the hall to the consultation room and begin to organize my few remaining papers and textbooks. Starting tomorrow, three thousand people will need to find a new doctor in a city that has six medical schools, but does not have enough primary care facilities, or general family-practice offices, or internal medicine clinics, or pediatric offices to provide access to medical care for the people who live in the community. Where my patients will go for their medical care, where the children I have taken care of will go for their immunizations, is unclear.

I look out the office window at the projects and at the empty lot across the street. I think of the Street Sound Bar, of Mr. Gregory, Marjeta Bradley, Ezekiel, and the others. I close my eyes for a moment, then turn and pack the last few books and papers. I open my briefcase, put in my stethoscope, then click the briefcase closed. It is time for me to go. I glance out the window. It is their home.